The AIDS Handbook

Third edition fully revised

**A guide to the prevention of
AIDS and HIV**

John Hubley BSc PhD

Consultant in international health education and health promotion
Senior Lecturer in Health Education and Health Promotion, Leeds
Metropolitan University, Leeds, United Kingdom

MACMILLAN

Macmillan Education
Between Towns Road, Oxford OX4 3PP
A division of Macmillan Publishers Limited
Companies and representatives throughout the world

www.macmillan-africa.com

ISBN - 13 : 978-0-333-94576-6
ISBN - 10 : 0-333-94576-X

Text © J.Hubley 2002
Design and illustration © Macmillan Publishers Limited 2002

First edition 1990
Reprinted twice
Second edition, fully revised 1995
Third edition, fully revised 2002

Typeset by Dave Glover
Cover design by Gary Fielder, AC Design
Cover photographs by John and Penny Hubley

Printed in Malaysia

2006
10 9 8 7 6 5 4

Contents

Preface

AIDS was the most important new threat to world health to emerge during the last century. In the absence of an affordable and effective cure or vaccine, health education directed at modifying risk behaviour is the only way in which the disease can be contained.

This aim of this book is to prepare those who are becoming involved in AIDS education in their family, community and workplace. It is also intended to meet the needs of those wishing a basic introduction to the disease and how to reduce the risk of becoming infected. The emphasis in the book is on the special needs of those working in developing countries. Particular attention is directed at describing the pattern of AIDS and role of AIDS education in developing countries.

The first priority for educating others is to learn about the disease ourselves so we can dispel the myths and rumours that surround AIDS and answer the searching questions that we will be asked by the community. The first four chapters will provide specific information on the disease, symptoms, extent of the problem, how it is transmitted. The factual chapters are followed by Chapter 5, which describes the actions to be take by communities to prevent the diseases and the role of UNAIDS and National AIDS Committees. Chapter 6 gives a brief review of counselling and its role in reducing risk behaviour and supporting those infected with HIV and AIDS. The final chapter provides guidelines on how to implement an action plan to run an AIDS education programme in your community.

I have attempted to steer a middle path. I have avoided providing an over-simplified description with insufficient detail to help you deal with questions you may be asked. On the other hand I have tried to avoid too detailed and academic a treatment of what is a complex and rapidly changing subject. With topics surrounded by controversy and debate, I have presented the current accepted view and have drawn heavily on discussions with the members of UNAIDS and their extensive series of technical memoranda. However, although some of the early experience on which this book is based was obtained while working as a consultant for the Global Programme on AIDS, this book represents my own views and not the official view of WHO or UNAIDS.

At points in this book I have provided the names of specific drugs that are currently used to treat both AIDS and opportunistic diseases. You should consult your own national guidelines for details of current recommendations and specific doses. Many of the medicines should only be given under the supervision of health workers who are trained in their use. In addition you should always check expiry dates on medicines and specific instructions provided.

For those who wish to read more about AIDS, counselling and educational methods I have included a short bibliography as well as a list of WHO technical reviews. I have also included details of newsletters that will keep you up to date on new developments in this fast-moving field. AIDS is a topic that is particularly well served on the Internet and I have included details of useful Web sites.

The stimulus for writing the book has been the expressed needs of my students at Leeds as well as participants on workshops and courses I have assisted in various countries in Africa. I would like to thank all of them for the ideas and suggestions that have contributed so much to this book.

John Hubley

Acknowledgements

I would like to thank the following for use of materials in this book: Brook Advisory Centres for leaflet on use of condoms; Teaching-aids At Low Cost for diagram on counselling. The GATHER model for counselling is adapted from the special issue of *Population Reports* on counselling produced by the Population Information Program of Johns Hopkins University. Reported cases of persons living with AIDS at end of 2000 is reproduced with permission of UNAIDS. The photograph of Lea Salonga by John Harris was selected from Photoshare, the online photo database of the Media/Materials Clearinghouse of the JHU/ Population Information Programme at www.jhuccp.org/mmc. My thanks to Dr Patrick Coleman and Lavinia Velasco for their help in selecting the photograph. The Female Health Company kindly provided the diagram of the female condom.

The portrayal of persons in photographs used in this book does not imply that they are HIV positive. They were chosen as positive images of communities taking action against AIDS. I would like to thank all those who appear in the photographs.

I would also like to thank the following for helpful suggestions on technical content of current and previous editions of this book: Dr Paul Sato, WHO GPA; Dr John Peabody and WHO Western Pacific Region; Elizabeth Preble, UNICEF New York. I would also like to thank: Dr Peter Fasan, Dr George Peterson and Dr John Peabody for their stimulating ideas during our WHO missions. Thanks also to Professor David Morley, Dr Felicity Savage King and Professor Andrew Tomkins for encouragement and ideas on the text and to Wendy Holmes for her thoughtful suggestions on counselling. I also would like to thank the Health Educators and AIDS activists in a number of countries where I have had the privilege of working with in AIDS and STD programmes: Dr Chandra Mouli (India and WHO, Geneva), Benjamin Binagwa (Uganda), Martha Osei (Ghana), Pitnera Mthembu (Swaziland), Mokuba Petlane (Lesotho), Winston Bomba, Elias Tsokolide and Paul Makhumula (Malawi) and Dr Qureshi Hyatt (Brunei). While the above have contributed in their different ways, the responsibility for the accuracy and content of the book is ultimately my own.

Like many, my early involvement in AIDS programmes was influenced and guided by the leadership of Dr Jonathan Mann, the first Director of the Global Programme on AIDS who was tragically killed in a plane crash in 1998. His contribution to the struggle against AIDS was enormous. I will miss him.

In writing the first two editions of this book I was inspired, encouraged and supported by my wife Penny. Her untimely death from breast cancer was a sad blow and this edition is dedicated to her memory.

1. Introduction

What is AIDS?

The full name for AIDS is Acquired Immune Deficiency Syndrome. As the name implies it is a disease caused by a deficiency in the body's immune system. It is a *syndrome* because there are a range of different symptoms that are not always found in each case. It is *acquired* because AIDS is an infectious disease caused by a virus that is spread from person to person through a variety of routes. This makes it different from immune deficiency from other causes such as treatment with anticancer drugs or immune system suppressing drugs given to persons receiving transplant operations.

History

AIDS is a new disease and some of the key dates in the discovery of the disease, cause and control are summarised below.

Timetable of important events in the history of AIDS

pre 1980 silent period: HIV being transmitted before AIDS was recognized as new disease

1981   Epidemic of *Pneumonocystis carinii* infection in Los Angeles, USA.
1981   Epidemic of Kaposi's sarcoma in New York, USA.
1982   Case definition produced for AIDS by Centers for Disease Control, Atlanta.
1982   Slim disease encountered in Rakai, Uganda.
1983   Increase in Kaposi's sarcoma found in Lusaka, Zambia.
1983   Isolation of HIV virus by Luc Montagnier in France.
1985   ELISA blood test developed.
1986   Dr Halfdan Mahler, then Director of WHO, addresses United Nations about AIDS.
1987   WHO Special Programme on AIDS formed becoming a Global Programme on AIDS in 1988.
1988   First global meeting of health ministers on AIDS.
1989   Red ribbon launched as international symbol of AIDS awareness.

1993	US Food and Drug Administration approves female condom.
1994	Paediatric AIDS Clinical Trials Group showed that treatment with AZT could reduce mother-to-infant transmission of HIV.
1995	Positive results emerge from first major trial of combination therapy (Delta trial).
1995	Intervention study in Mwanza, Tanzania establishes that treatment of sexually transmitted diseases will prevent HIV transmission.
1996	Joint United Nations programme on AIDS – UNAIDS – became operational.
1996	Global AIDS vaccine initiative launched.
1997	Human rights guidelines from Second International Consultation on HIV/AIDS and Human Rights.
1998	14 members of Southern African Develoment Community (SADC) adopt policy for AIDS in the workplace.
2000	UN Security Council holds its first ever meeting concerning a health issue: HIV and AIDS.

How did it begin?

In 1981 doctors in Los Angeles found themselves baffled by a strange disease. Apparently healthy young men were developing pneumonia caused by a microorganism *Pneumocystis carinii* which does not usually cause the disease in normal healthy persons. This unusual infection had previously been found only in persons whose immune systems had been weakened as a result of treatment with powerful medicines (such as anticancer agents or immunosuppressant agents). Besides *Pneumocystis carinii* these men were suffering from a range of other 'opportunistic infections', which healthy persons should normally be able to resist.

In 1981 doctors in New York came across another puzzling disease in young men. This was a rare skin cancer called Kaposi's sarcoma that had also been previously only reported in people with damaged immune systems.

Researchers found that the young men were all homosexuals, many of whom were also suffering from sexually transmitted diseases such as gonorrhoea and syphilis. It was thought likely that this new disease was also a sexually transmitted disease.

These symptoms were then found in other sections of the population who were not homosexuals – haemophiliacs and persons injecting drugs such as heroin. Haemophilia is an inherited disease where the blood lacks the essential factors needed for clotting and healing of wounds. These persons were receiving injections of a substance called Factor 8 made from blood of healthy persons without haemophilia. Many of the injecting drug users did not sterilise their needles and shared them with other addicts. It became clear to the researchers that not only was AIDS a sexually transmitted disease but it could also be transmitted through blood.

By 1982 the Centers for Disease Control in Atlanta, United States decided that enough was known about the disease to produce a provisional case definition. AIDS was defined as the presence of reliably defined diseases that are due to an underlying immune deficiency, e.g. *Pneumocystis carinii* pneumonia or Kaposi's sarcoma and also where the immune deficiency is not due to other known causes such as congenital diseases, immunosuppressant drugs or cancer.

In Africa, doctors were also coming across patients with unusual symptoms. In Kigali in Rwanda and Kinshasha in Zaire there was in 1980 an increase in the disease cryptococcal meningitis. In Rakai district in Uganda, a disease was found where young people dramatically lost weight and died. This became known as 'slim disease'. In 1983, this same wasting disease was reported in Zambia together with Kaposi's sarcoma. It seemed likely that these diseases in Africa were the same as this new disease AIDS in USA.

In 1983 Luc Montagnier from the Pasteur Institute in France isolated a virus from the blood of AIDS patients which he called Lymphadenopathy Associated Virus or LAV. In 1984 Robert Gallo and his fellow workers at the National Cancer Institute in the United States isolated a virus that they called the Human T cell Lymphotrophic Virus or HTLV III. These two viruses were shown to be the same and in 1986 an international committee agreed to rename the virus as Human Immunodeficiency Virus or HIV. Further work has shown there to be at least one other virus capable of producing the signs and symptoms AIDS. The original virus has been called HIV1 and the second one HIV2. A fuller account of the biology of the different viruses is given in Chapter 2.

Once the virus was isolated it became possible to develop tests to detect antibodies to the virus in blood. One of the early tests was the ELISA test (see Chapter 2 for a fuller account of tests). It became possible to carry out surveys of different groups of the public and determine different levels of infection with the virus.

It was found that there could be a period of up to 10 years between being infected with the virus and developing the symptoms of AIDS. For each person with symptoms of AIDS there could be more than 100 others who were carrying the virus but did not have the disease. These 'HIV antibody positive persons' – sometimes called 'HIV positive', 'seropositive' or 'carriers' – showed no signs of AIDS at that point in time but were able to infect others.

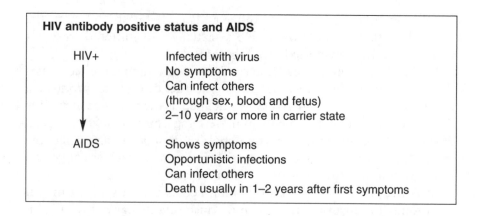

HIV antibody positive status and AIDS

HIV+   Infected with virus
        No symptoms
        Can infect others
        (through sex, blood and fetus)
        2–10 years or more in carrier state

AIDS   Shows symptoms
        Opportunistic infections
        Can infect others
        Death usually in 1–2 years after first symptoms

In 1987 the member nations of the World Health Organization (WHO) recognised the seriousness of the emerging AIDS epidemic by creating a special programme that in 1988 became the Global Programme on AIDS. This became the focal point for an intense international effort to develop comprehensive national plans for the prevention and control of AIDS. It soon became clear that control of the AIDS epidemic went well beyond health issues to encompass social, political and economic areas of life. In recognition of this, in 1996 the United Nations set up UNAIDS to provide the global leadership to take the struggle against AIDS into the twenty-first century.

The size of the problem – global level

At the end of the twentieth century

- Over 14,000 new HIV infections a day occurred in the year 2000.
- More than 95% of these are in developing countries.
- 1600 are in children under 15 years of age.
- Over half of the infected adults are under 25 years.
- 5.3 million new infections over whole year.
- Total number of people living with HIV/AIDS 36.1 million.
- Deaths due to HIV/AIDS in 2000 3 million – of which 500,000 were children.
- Total deaths due to HIV/AIDS since the beginning of the epidemic 21.8 million.

By the end of the twentieth century AIDS had spread to all continents and most countries – the disease is *pandemic*.

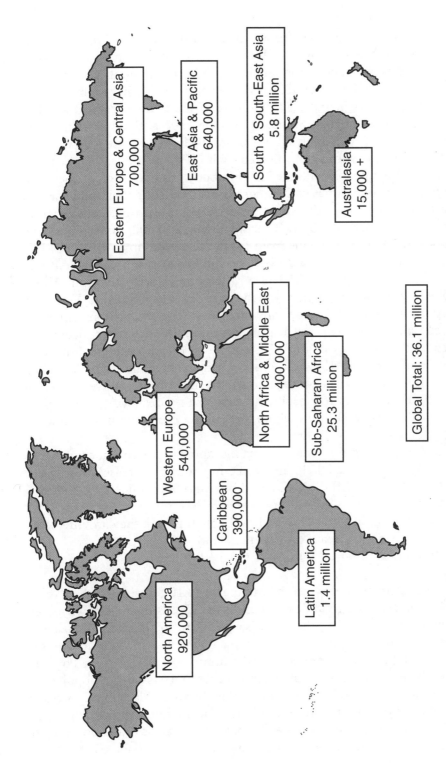

Figure 1. Adults and children estimated to be living with HIV/AIDS as of end 2000 (UNAIDS)

Eastern Europe & Central Asia
700,000

East Asia & Pacific
640,000

South & South-East Asia
5.8 million

Australasia
15,000 +

North Africa & Middle East
400,000

Sub-Saharan Africa
25.3 million

Global Total: 36.1 million

Western Europe
540,000

Caribbean
390,000

North America
920,000

Latin America
1.4 million

Only a few years ago tuberculosis (TB) was a disease that was thought to be under control. However, tuberculosis can be activated by HIV and is showing a dramatic increase in many countries. Around 8 million people become sick with TB each year. Of these 3 million are in South-East Asia and 1.5 million are in sub-Saharan Africa, which is facing a massive rise. Someone who is HIV antibody positive and infected with TB is many times more likely to become sick with TB than someone who is not infected with HIV. TB is a leading cause of death among people who are HIV antibody positive. Poorly supervised treatment programmes with patients not completing their full course of treatment has made the situation even worse with the emergence of multi-drug resistant TB. WHO estimate that 200 million people will get sick and 70 million will die from TB in the period up to the year 2020. At least one in six of these TB cases will be the result of HIV/AIDS.

Most countries provide data on the number of deaths from AIDS, which give an indication of the size of the problem. However, reporting of deaths, especially in remote rural locations, may be incomplete. Even when a death is reported, the death certificate may report the cause of death as tuberculosis, diarrhoea or malnutrition and not mention AIDS as the underlying cause. The stigma attached to AIDS can also encourage the reporting of alternative causes of death. Because of these problems, reported figures for AIDS are often lower than the real levels which, depending on the country, could be much higher.

Even allowing for under-reporting, knowing the number of AIDS deaths is of limited help in predicting future increases. For every reported case of AIDS there could be up to 5000 infected persons:

- showing no symptoms and probably unaware they are infected;
- passing the disease on to others; and
- who will be the AIDS cases for the future.

The distinction between the numbers of AIDS cases and the level of infection causes a great deal of confusion. This is the reason why, even now, many people deny that there is a problem. To obtain a more realistic estimate of the size of the problem in a country, we need to look at the level of HIV *infection* rather than the number of AIDS cases. This can only be estimated from conducting antibody tests on the population. This has not always been possible, either because of lack of resources or public opposition. The need to obtain information for planning AIDS prevention programmes has to be balanced against the importance of safeguarding human rights of persons found to be infected.

Results from testing have to be treated with some caution because they may not be representative of the whole population. Ideally these should be 'sero-surveys' of representative samples of the country's population. When sero-surveys are not possible, it is necessary to rely on testing samples of blood that have been drawn for other reasons such as from blood donors or women presenting themselves at antenatal clinics. Data from these sources may not give a true picture. For example in India paid blood donors have a higher level of HIV infection than voluntary donors. The women who attend antenatal clinics are not typical of the general population as HIV infection can reduce a woman's chance of becoming pregnant.

Another source of information on the extent of infection in the community comes from studies of antibody levels in special groups of the public who are seen as particularly at risk. These might be sex workers (prostitutes) or patients at clinics for sexually transmitted diseases.

The early tests developed in western countries were not very reliable in Africa and produced many 'false positives'. This led to scares and suspicion that AIDS was being grossly exaggerated by the West who were putting the blame on Africa. However, tests developed since then have greatly improved and highly specific confirmatory tests have been developed (see Chapter 2). Levels of infections as high as 10–25% and even more in the urban sexually active age groups have been found in the worst affected countries.

Figure 1 shows the numbers of people estimated by UNAIDS to be living with AIDS at the end of 2000. This includes both persons infected with HIV and showing symptoms of AIDS. This estimate has been produced by taking into account reported AIDS cases and the results of sero-surveys. Different regions have different numbers of people and it is useful to express the data as prevalence – the proportion of the population living with HIV/AIDS. According to UNAIDS at the end of the year 2000 the prevalence rate of HIV/AIDS among adults aged 15–49 years in the world was 1.1%. However, this figure concealed wide variations with the prevalence level of sub-Saharan Africa the greatest at 8.8%, Caribbean 2.3%, South and South-East Asia 0.56%, North America 0.6% and Western Europe 0.24%.

The global distribution of AIDS and HIV

A question that is frequently asked is why levels of HIV infection are less in some countries than others. The reason for the lower prevalence of HIV infection in some countries such as the Middle East, China and the Pacific is probably an accident of time. By the time the infection reached these regions and countries the world was aware of AIDS and the routes by which HIV was transmitted and could be controlled. However, the situation in a country can change rapidly (see below the example of the Russian Republic). Without continued effort at control, it is only a question of time before levels reach those of high prevalence countries.

In **The United States, Europe and Australasia** HIV began to spread extensively from the late 1970s and early 1980s. Initially the United States had the World's highest numbers of reported AIDS cases. Most of the people affected were homosexual and bisexual men, injecting drug users and their sex partners. The incidence of new cases of HIV among homosexual men declined as a result of the impact of educational programmes. However, HIV incidence among drug injectors and heterosexuals is still increasing.

The levels of HIV infection in **Eastern Europe and Central Asia, including the former Soviet Union** are low but increasing rapidly. The proportion of people living with HIV doubled between 1997 and 1999 and doubled again during the year 2000. Most of these of new HIV infections were caused by unsafe injection of drugs in just two countries, the Russian Republic and Ukraine.

In **sub-Saharan Africa**, the situation is particularly serious and the region has the highest level of people living with HIV and AIDS. Transmission has been mainly through heterosexual sex, mother-to-child routes with some spread through blood transfusions. While in Europe and North America the disease burden of AIDS has mainly fallen on men, in sub-Saharan Africa it is women and their babies who are the most affected.

- Overall 55% of infected adults in sub-Saharan Africa are women, which means more than six HIV positive women for every five HIV positive men. UNAIDS and WHO estimate that 25.3 million people in sub-Saharan Africa are living with HIV at the end of 2000.
- Four out of five HIV positive women in the world live in Africa.
- Recent studies reviewed by UNAIDS in several African populations found that girls aged 15–19 are around five or six times more likely to be HIV positive than boys their own age. This is probably due to practices such as 'sugar daddies' where older men buy sexual favours from young girls.
- Nine out every ten babies infected through their mothers are in Africa.

While originally concentrated in urban areas, infection spread to rural areas. The early epidemic closely followed the highways, with truck drivers and roadside night stops playing a significant role in transmission.

In recent years the burden of HIV/AIDS has shifted to Southern Africa – especially South Africa – where the large numbers of men away from home working in mines has encouraged rapid spread of HIV. With the exception of Côte d'Ivoire, prevalence of HIV/AIDS in West Africa is lower than other parts of the region. However, even with the lower prevalence, Nigeria's large population of over 100 million will result in an estimated 2 million people living with HIV and AIDS, a major burden on already stretched health and social services.

A ray of hope in Africa is provided by Uganda where recent studies suggest that HIV infection among young persons is showing some decline and sexual behaviours are changing. Unlike most countries where denial and delay were the norm, Uganda was one of the first countries in Africa to accept that it had a problem and mobilise for action (see the booklet *Open Secret* in the Strategies of Hope series referred to at the end of this book for a fuller description of Uganda's open policy).

In **Asia and the Pacific** HIV was first recognised in 1985 in Thailand. In most other Asian countries HIV was not diagnosed until 1986 or later. But since then, HIV has spread rapidly and has been found in most of the countries. In Thailand, in early 1990, there were over 50,000 infected persons. By late 1992 WHO estimated the number had risen *by nine times* to 450,000. UNAIDS estimates that about 3.7 million persons in India are infected with HIV. The size of the epidemic in the other giant of Asia, China, is still comparatively low with almost half a million people in a population of 1000 million estimated to be HIV positive – mainly through injecting drug use. Drug injection has played a major role in the initial spread of HIV in Thailand, Myanmar and north-east India. The other main mode of transmission is heterosexual sex.

The infections acquired through needle-sharing have spread through heterosexual sex to other adults. Commercial sex work (prostitution) is also playing a major role in spreading HIV. Some countries such as Thailand and the Philippines are visited by tourists, usually men, wishing to have sex for money with other men, women and even children – so called 'sex tourism'.

The emergence of the AIDS epidemic in Asia has brought homosexuality into the open. Many countries are recognising that AIDS cannot be controlled without measures which protect the rights of homosexuals.

The vigorous AIDS prevention campaigns in Thailand make it one of the few countries where the increase in levels of HIV infection has slowed down. During the 1990s studies have shown reductions in prevalence of HIV infections among military conscripts and pregnant women. This is likely to be due to changes in sexual behaviour including use of condoms.

Another note of optimism comes from the Philippines where levels of HIV infection have remained low. UNAIDS suggests that this is due to an enlightened government policy in which prostitutes are registered, screened every 2 weeks for other sexually transmitted infections and report a high level of condom use.

Levels of AIDS and HIV infection in the Pacific Islands are still low. However, the levels of sexually transmitted diseases and the high mobility of these small island populations suggest that HIV will spread rapidly and have a major impact on these fragile island economies (as has already happened in the Caribbean – see below).

In **North Africa and the Middle East:** Less is known of the true extent of the epidemic in this region. UNAIDS estimates that at the end of 2000 there were 400,000 adults and children living with HIV and AIDS. Extensive spread of HIV only began in the late 1980s and the main route is sexual transmission and injecting drug use.

Latin America and the Caribbean: As of the end of 2000 UNAIDS estimates 1.8 million persons living with HIV and AIDS, with Brazil having the most reported cases. In South America the number of infections is greatest in homosexual and bisexual men, but transmission among heterosexuals and drug injectors is increasing. The numbers of persons with AIDS in the Caribbean appear low but this is deceptive. When their small populations are taken into account, the Caribbean islands have the second highest prevalence rate for HIV/AIDS after Africa.

AIDS and development

AIDS has had a devastating effect on individuals, families and communities everywhere the disease has spread. However, it is the developing countries of the Caribbean, Latin America, Asia and sub-Saharan Africa where the situation is most worrying and the AIDS epidemic will have a major impact on their already severe problems.

At the *individual and family level* AIDS leads to:

- loss of income-earning opportunities because of sickness and the need to care for the sick;
- money being diverted away from food, schools and other household expenditures to pay for medical costs, funeral expenses and caring for orphans;
- withdrawal of children from school to reduce expenditure and increase labour;
- stigmatisation, prejudice and persecution of people with AIDS and HIV.

> **At the *national level* AIDS is having an impact on development through:**
> - loss of productive trained labour reducing productivity of key industries;
> - money being diverted from other health issues to treatment of AIDS patients.

With the world's highest levels of HIV and AIDS, it is sub-Saharan Africa where the social and economic impact will be greatest. A report from the World Bank in 1999 describes the crisis ahead:

> Tragically mass killers are nothing new in Africa. Malaria still claims about as many African lives as AIDS and preventable childhood diseases kill millions of others. What sets AIDS apart, however, is its unprecedented impact on regional development. Because it kills so many adults in the prime of their working and parenting lives, it decimates the workforce, fractures and impoverishes families, orphans millions, and shreds the fabric of communities.

Reviews by UNAIDS provide grim examples of the impact that AIDS is having on education, social and health services. Treatment of AIDS is estimated to take up 39% of the beds in Kenyatta National Hospital in Nairobi, Kenya; over a quarter of the health spending in Zimbabwe; and two-thirds that of Rwanda. In the first 10 months of 1998 Zambia lost 1300 teachers because of AIDS – equivalent to two-thirds of their annual output from teacher training colleges.

The serious economic and social impact of AIDS was shown in a study reviewed by UNAIDS of commercial farms in Kenya. In one sugar estate one in four of the workforce was infected with HIV. Between 1989 and 1997 there was an increase in absenteeism, company spending on funerals increased fivefold, expenditure on health provision increased tenfold and productivity declined.

In many countries, rural poverty has led to migration and a rapid expansion of the cities. In these growing cities social problems have arisen such as unemployment, slums/shanty townships, prostitution and 'street children'. In some countries political upheavals and wars have led to a refugee crisis. Traditional stable family structures have come under pressure and norms of sexual behaviour are changing.

Developing countries do not have the resources and infrastructure of health services, communication media and trained field staff that industrialised countries are able to draw on for mounting public education campaigns, blood screening programmes and for treatment of AIDS patients. A *vicious circle* is emerging: poverty and social upheaval are underlying factors in the spread of HIV; the resulting AIDS epidemic is causing further social and economic distress at all levels of society. In response to the seriousness of the AIDS epidemic, the Security Council of the United Nations met in January 2000 for the first ever time to discuss AIDS. At that meeting Kofi Annan, Secretary General of the United Nations, told the Council that the '... impact of AIDS is no less destructive than that of warfare itself, and by some measures, far worse'.

The cost of doing nothing

The cost of inaction will be great. The already high burden of AIDS faced by many countries is only the 'tip of the iceberg'. Many of these people with HIV will develop clinical symptoms of AIDS over the next few years, take up hospital beds and use up health resources.

Life expectancy at birth in Southern Africa made impressive gains from 44 years in the early 1950s to 59 years in the early 1990s. AIDS will reverse the beneficial impact of these public health programmes and UNAIDS predicts that life expectancy will drop back to the levels of the 1950s. Already in parts of Africa deaths of children from AIDS are overshadowing the gains that had been made through primary health care and immunisation. The lesson is clear, action is needed *now*!

A sustained, coordinated programme is needed to deal with HIV and AIDS in all countries. *Everyone*, both professional and lay, has a role to play in these programmes. This book is intended to provide the necessary background information that will enable you to undertake health education in your family, community and workplace. It includes chapters on the virus, symptoms, treatment, transmission, prevention, counselling and planning health education programmes. Inevitably I have had to simplify some of the technical issues and there is a list of books and Internet sites for those who wish to read further.

2. The biology of the virus

The Human Immunodeficiency Virus (HIV)

A virus is an infectious particle that is too small to be seen with the naked eye or even a conventional light microscope. Bacteria are 1/1000 of a millimetre and can be seen with a light microscope. A virus such as HIV is 1/10,000 of a millimetre in diameter and can only be seen with an electron microscope.

Evidence for the role of HIV in causing AIDS comes from the following:

- HIV has been detected in persons with AIDS.
- People who develop AIDS are those who were HIV antibody positive or who have been shown to carry the virus.
- HIV has been shown to infect cells in the immune system so the role of HIV in causing AIDS makes biological sense.

Strong evidence for the role of HIV also came from a detailed follow-up study of 7800 people in Masaka District of Uganda whose findings were reported in 1993. The research team found that the risk of dying during a one-year period was 60 times higher for persons infected with HIV than for persons who were not infected. Another powerful argument for HIV came from study of twins of HIV-infected mothers. In situations when one twin is infected with HIV and the other it is not, it is the baby with HIV that develops AIDS and the other is normal.

A diagram of the HIV virus which causes AIDS is shown in Figure 2. It has a very simple structure consisting of an outer coat or envelope made up of a lipid membrane with two kinds of special molecules called glycoproteins labelled GP-120 and GP-41. This outer coat covers a core made up of proteins labelled P-24 and P-17.

Inside the core is located the genetic material containing the information needed for the virus to reproduce itself. Most viruses have

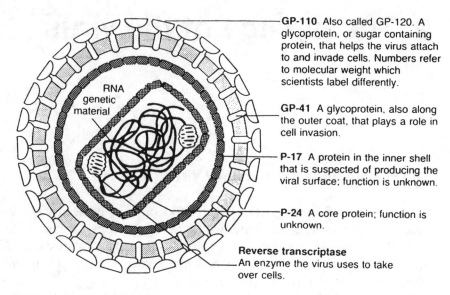

GP-110 Also called GP-120. A glycoprotein, or sugar containing protein, that helps the virus attach to and invade cells. Numbers refer to molecular weight which scientists label differently.

GP-41 A glycoprotein, also along the outer coat, that plays a role in cell invasion.

P-17 A protein in the inner shell that is suspected of producing the viral surface; function is unknown.

P-24 A core protein; function is unknown.

Reverse transcriptase An enzyme the virus uses to take over cells.

RNA genetic material

Figure 2. Human Immunodeficiency Virus

genetic material made up of DNA. However HIV belongs to an unusual class of viruses called *retroviruses* where the genetic material is in the form of RNA.

Unlike bacteria, viruses cannot reproduce themselves outside a living cell. When they infect a person they enter the cells of the host. HIV recognises and is able to attach itself to a molecule called CD4 on the wall of the T4 lymphocyte cell. As shown in Figure 3, they are able to direct the biological machinery of the host cell to make new virus particles that can be released to infect other cells. Retroviruses also contain a highly unusual enzyme called reverse transcriptase. This enzyme is able to convert the viral RNA into DNA. This DNA is then incorporated into the genes of the host cell. When the host cell replicates itself, the virus DNA will also be copied. The virus will stay in the host cell and cannot be eliminated. At a later stage, some event, which is not well understood by scientists, triggers the host T4 cells to produce HIV viruses.

Viruses cause many infections such as measles, mumps and colds. The human body has a very efficient defence mechanism to protect against infection by viruses and other germs. This 'immune defence system' operates by the production of antibodies that destroy the virus. The unique feature of HIV, which makes it so dangerous, is that the part of our body that it attacks is cells vital to the body's immune defence.

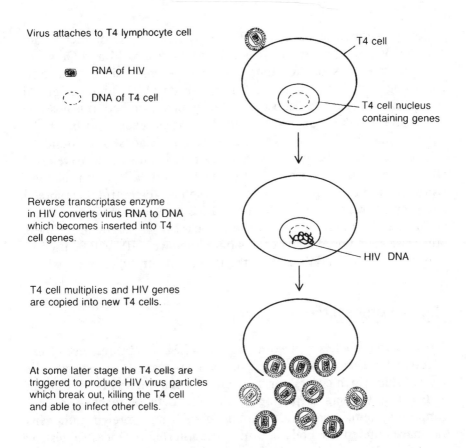

Virus attaches to T4 lymphocyte cell

RNA of HIV

DNA of T4 cell

T4 cell

T4 cell nucleus containing genes

Reverse transcriptase enzyme in HIV converts virus RNA to DNA which becomes inserted into T4 cell genes.

HIV DNA

T4 cell multiplies and HIV genes are copied into new T4 cells.

At some later stage the T4 cells are triggered to produce HIV virus particles which break out, killing the T4 cell and able to infect other cells.

Figure 3. Replication of Human Immunodeficiency Virus (HIV)

These cells are called the 'T4 lymphocytes'. Figure 3 shows how HIV attacks these T4 lymphocytes. The HIV virus is deadly because it strips our bodies of their defence systems.

HIV was discovered in 1983 and has since been found worldwide. In 1987 a similar virus was discovered in West Africa. This newer virus was called HIV2 and the original virus named HIV1. HIV2 has been mainly found in West Africa but, as people travel, is beginning to spread to other parts of Africa, Asia and Europe.

While the chemical and genetic structure of HIV2 is similar to HIV1, there are differences. Both are retroviruses and appear to affect the immune system in a similar manner through attacking the T4 lymphocytes. Both viruses appear to produce similar clinical symptoms, which take longer to develop in persons infected with HIV2. Both HIV1 and HIV2 are transmitted in the same way through blood and sex and mother to child. However, it is thought that HIV2 is not transmitted as easily as HIV1 especially by the mother to her child. HIV1 can be further divided into two groups M and O, which in turn can be separated into sub-types – also called 'clades' – according to their chemical and genetic structure. The implications of these different types and sub-types are still being studied. It is possible that some may be more easily spread by homosexual and others by heterosexual intercourse. The sub-types or 'clades' are found in different parts of the world with some more common in developed and others in developing countries. HIV2 and HIV1, and all their types and sub-types, require the same response to control their spread and prevent transmission. Where the differences become important is in the development of vaccines and possibly in treatment. Unless otherwise stated, in the rest of this book the term HIV will be used to refer to HIV1 and HIV2 and all the types and sub-types.

The immune system

The human body has evolved many mechanisms to protect itself from infection by disease-causing microorganisms (called pathogens). The layer of skin which covers our body and the acid juices in the stomach both act as barriers to pathogens. A third defence mechanism, the immune system, involves the ability to recognise foreign pathogens that have entered the body and mobilise internal defences to destroy them. The body is also able to remember the characteristics of the pathogen, so that next time the body is invaded by that microorganism it is able to respond even quicker. This last property of memory is drawn on when we produce vaccines for immunisation against diseases such as polio, measles and yellow fever.

We are continually coming into contact with microorganisms every time we eat food, breath air or injure ourselves. The immune system is constantly vigilant and most invasions of pathogens are successfully dealt with by our immune system without us even being aware of it. It is thanks to our immune system that only a few types of microorganisms are able to cause disease.

The HIV virus is unique and deadly because it attacks a key group of cells in the body called T4 lymphocytes that coordinate the body's immune defence system. This prevents the body from mobilising effectively against the HIV virus. More importantly, it leaves the body open to infection from a wide range of microorganisms which do not normally cause serious illness in persons with functioning immune systems.

Some further details of the immune system

This section is a highly simplified summary of the complex mechanism by which the different components of the immune system work together to destroy invading disease-causing organisms. You should only read it if you feel that you are likely to be asked detailed questions by others and need this specialist knowledge.

Those components of an organism that stimulate an immune response are called *antigens*. The word antigen is a general term for a molecule, on its own or part of a disease-causing organism, which is capable of reacting with the immune system and stimulating an immune response.

There are two main systems through which the immune defence system operates. The first type, called *humoral immunity*, is based on the production of large molecules called antibodies which circulate in a person's blood. These molecules are produced when the body is invaded by foreign substances. Antigens stimulate the production of antibodies by cells called B lymphocytes. The antibodies produced by the body in response to this foreign invasion are able to attach themselves specifically to the foreign substances which are then inactivated by other cells called 'killer T cells'. This sequence is shown as follows.

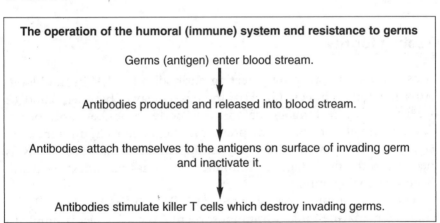

The operation of the humoral (immune) system and resistance to germs

Germs (antigen) enter blood stream.

↓

Antibodies produced and released into blood stream.

↓

Antibodies attach themselves to the antigens on surface of invading germ and inactivate it.

↓

Antibodies stimulate killer T cells which destroy invading germs.

As well as the mechanism of defence described above based on antibody molecules in the blood, there is a second type that is based on a group of specialised cells in the immune system. This system is called *cell-mediated immunity*.

When a disease-causing microorganism enters the body, a group of cells called macrophages are usually the first to respond. They ingest the pathogen and present the antigens on it to an important type of cell called the T4 lymphocyte. These T4 cells are also called 'Helper T Cells' because they stimulate the production of antibodies by the humoral system described above as well as several other functions that are described below. HIV affects all these important functions in the immune system when it infects and destroys these important T4 lymphocytes.

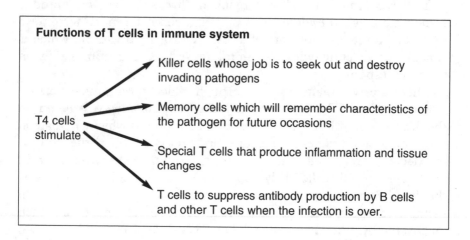

Functions of T cells in immune system

T4 cells stimulate

Killer cells whose job is to seek out and destroy invading pathogens

Memory cells which will remember characteristics of the pathogen for future occasions

Special T cells that produce inflammation and tissue changes

T cells to suppress antibody production by B cells and other T cells when the infection is over.

Testing for HIV

Most AIDS tests work by detecting antibodies to HIV in the blood. After the body is infected by HIV there is a delay of between 3 and 12 weeks (or even longer) before the body produces antibodies. Antibodies will continue to be present in the blood right until the final stages of AIDS when they may disappear in some cases. This is because in the final stage the immune system has been destroyed and is not producing antibodies.

The most common screening test for HIV is the ELISA test. ELISA stands for Enzyme Linked Immunosorbent Assay. The test is simple to carry out by trained laboratory workers and costs about US$1–2. The test is very sensitive and will detect virtually all samples with HIV antibodies.

When evaluating HIV antibody tests it is useful to consider the following points:

- **False positives** are test results which indicate the presence of HIV antibodies when they are not there.

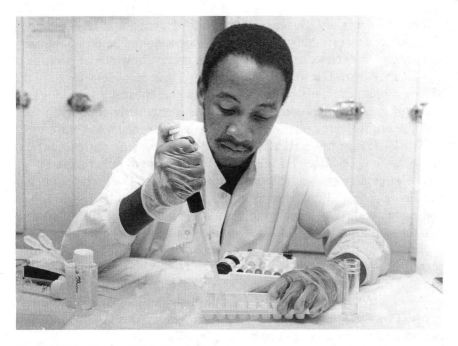

Figure 4. Testing for HIV antibodies

- **False negatives** are test results which find a negative result – i.e. no HIV antibodies – when there are antibodies present.
- A **specific** test is one which will only give a positive result with HIV antibodies and gives very few false positives. The specificity of a test is the probability that all the samples that a test shows to be positive are genuinely positive.
- A **sensitive** test will detect every sample with HIV antibodies and give very few false negatives. The sensitivity of a test is the probability that the test will only give a negative result with a sample that is genuinely negative.

Early versions of the ELISA test produced some false positives. In particular, the tests developed originally for use in Europe or USA gave high levels of false positives with blood samples from Africa. However, if used properly newer tests are more specific with very few false positives.

It is important to be really certain that a person is actually HIV antibody positive. This is because labelling a person as being infected with HIV has serious implications for the individual and is always traumatic. We cannot afford to make a mistake and subject a person to unnecessary anxiety. Because of the risk of occasional false positives many countries, especially where the prevalence of infection is low, carry out a supplementary test on each sample that is shown to be positive in the ELISA test. The supplementary test that is widely used is the Western blot test. This test measures the presence of antibodies to a series of specific virus coat proteins. This is expensive (about US$30) and difficult to carry out so it is only done at special test centres.

The ELISA and Western blot tests do not measure the presence of virus but the presence of antibodies. Antibodies are only formed 3–12 weeks after a person is infected with the virus. The period when a person is infected but has not produced detectable antibodies is sometimes called a 'window period'. During this window period a person could have HIV and be capable of infecting others but appear negative on the test. This has important implications for blood transfusion services as blood could be tested and certified free of HIV but still be infectious. It also explains why testing people on entering into a country is not a helpful control measure. People might appear negative on the test because they were tested during this window period and had not yet developed antibodies.

There are some problems with HIV antibody tests. Many tests such as the ELISA and Western blot can only be done at centres where there are trained laboratory staff, well-maintained equipment and a steady power supply. They can take 3 hours or more to get the results so are not suitable for emergencies such as when an accident victim requires blood urgently and there is no tested blood available in the blood bank. It is also important that the test kits are genuine and not fakes, that they have been stored according to the manufacturer's instructions (some may require refrigeration) and not passed their expiry dates.

Much effort has been put into research and evaluation of new tests that are quicker and do not require expensive equipment or extensive training. 'Rapid' tests are defined as those that can take 10 minutes and 'simple' tests are those that take longer. They are especially useful in emergency situations or as part of a voluntary counselling programme when a test result can be supplied on the same day (see Chapter 6). Unfortunately these simple/rapid tests can be more expensive and the test kits may need to be stored in a refrigerator.

Most tests are carried out on plasma (also called serum). A sample of blood has to be taken from the person and the red blood cells have to be removed by centrifuge to leave the plasma. Tests are being developed that can use whole blood, dried blood, urine or even saliva. However, the tests are not as specific and need a complementary test to confirm the result.

There are other kinds of tests that are very expensive and mainly used for research but might become cheaper in the future. These are *antigen tests* which measure the presence of the virus rather than antibodies. The polymerase chain reaction (PCR) test uses enzymes to copy and multiply the fragments of viral RNA until there is enough to be measured.

Origins of HIV and AIDS

The origin of the HIV viruses is only just beginning to be understood. During the early stages of the AIDS epidemic the flimsiest evidence was used to blame AIDS on Haitians and Africans. Justifiably, there was a strong reaction from African nations to the racism shown in many of these early pronouncements.

It is interesting to place AIDS in a historical perspective. When the disease syphilis ravaged Europe from the sixteenth century, that disease was also blamed on others. In Britain it was called the 'French disease'. With something new, strange and deadly there is an unfortunate tendency to blame it on other people. Wild unproven speculation about HIV having escaped from a germ warfare laboratory has not been helpful.

The theory that is increasingly accepted is that the virus was present in an animal where it did not cause disease and in some way was transferred to humans where it caused disease. There are several diseases that have animal carriers such as Lassa fever and plague. In 1999 a group of researchers from the University of Alabama announced that they had found a virus almost identical to HIV-1 in a sub-group of chimpanzees called *Pan troglodytes troglodytes* which were once common in West-Central Africa. Most researchers accept that this is the origin of HIV1. HIV2 is very similar to the Simian Immunodeficiency Virus (SIV) found in the sooty mangabey monkey (also called green monkey). There remains the question of how did the virus pass on to humans. It has been suggested that HIV might have been introduced by immunization campaigns in Zaire in the late 1950s which used polio vaccines derived from monkey tissue. However, there is no evidence to support that theory (and current polio vaccines are completely safe). A more likely explanation is that that HIV could have crossed over from chimpanzees as a result of a human killing a chimpanzee and eating it for food.

There has been continued speculation about other possible origins. However, whatever the origins, the unique features of the late twentieth century – internal migration, air travel, sexual freedom, blood transfusions and intravenous drug injectors all combined to spread the virus and create an epidemic of global proportions. The debate about the origins of AIDS has not been helpful because it has created bitterness and diverted attention from the important task of prevention. Kenneth Kaunda, the former President of Zambia, expressed it well when he said 'It is not important to know were it came from but rather where it is going!'

3. Symptoms and disease

Who is affected?

A typical distribution of AIDS patients by age in an African country is shown in Figure 5. This shows that AIDS is found mainly in the sexually active age group and the level among the very young or old is low. The large number of cases in the first 2 years is due to transmission of the virus from mother to the baby in the womb. The age range from 3 to 13 years has very little AIDS. The main source of infection for these children is likely to be contaminated blood transfusions.

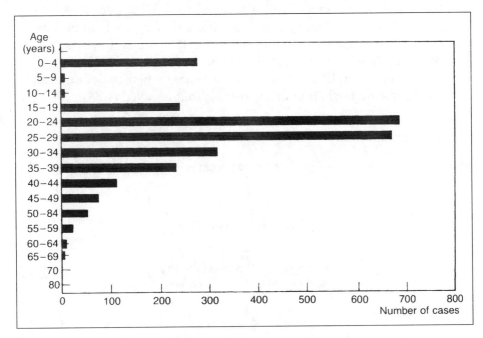

Figure 5. A typical distribution of reported AIDS cases in an African country

Symptoms and disease progression

Because AIDS is a syndrome, the symptoms can vary between individuals. Although the effect of HIV in damaging the immune system is the same in all countries, the actual pattern of symptoms can be different according to the opportunistic infections that are locally prevalent. For example pneumonia from *Pneumocystis carinii* and *Mycobacterium avium* complex disease (MAC) are found in Europe and USA but are less common in Africa. In Africa tuberculosis is a common opportunistic infection associated with AIDS but is less common in Europe.

Many of the symptoms described below (such as diarrhoea, weight loss, swollen lymph nodes) are not very specific. They often occur in people who do not have AIDS. Also, the nature and mix of symptoms can vary between countries. Hence, locally specific case definitions have been developed. Diagnosis should be done by trained health workers and should be based both on symptoms and the demonstration of the presence of HIV antibodies in the blood.

There has been a great deal of panic about AIDS. Because of the non-specific nature of many symptoms it is easy for people to become frightened and imagine that they have AIDS. It is important to counsel people who become anxious that they may have AIDS.

A number of conditions can be developed by a person before he or she develops the final stage of the disease that is called AIDS.

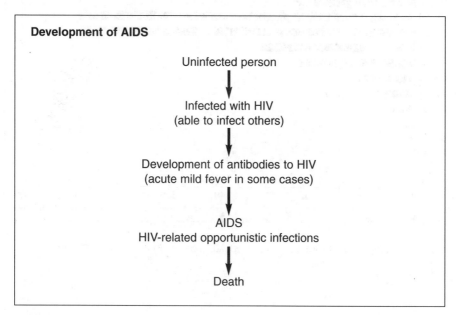

Development of AIDS

Uninfected person

Infected with HIV
(able to infect others)

Development of antibodies to HIV
(acute mild fever in some cases)

AIDS
HIV-related opportunistic infections

Death

After a person has been infected with the virus there is a period between 3 to 12 weeks before the body responds by the production of antibodies. During this period some people may experience a short bout of fever that is believed to accompany the production of antibodies. Right from the time of infection the person is in the *carrier* state, free of symptoms but capable of passing the virus to other persons.

It is thought that, eventually, all HIV antibody positive persons will go on to develop AIDS but the time taken to do this will vary from person to person. The factors that determine the rate of disease progression are not well understood but probably include the natural variation in resistance of hosts, other host factors including age and also variation in pathogenicity of different strains of HIV. The time taken for infected babies to progress to AIDS is short and most will have died by 5 years of age. With adults it can be around 7–10 years or even longer. WHO estimate that 50% of those infected become ill within 10 years of initial infection. Once a person develops AIDS, the average survival time is between 1 and 3 years. Less is known about HIV-2 infections. Evidence suggests that people infected with HIV-2 progress to AIDS more slowly than those with HIV-1. Studies suggest that the rate of progression to AIDS is faster in developing countries. This may be because people in these countries are much more exposed to common infectious diseases.

Symptoms

The symptoms of AIDS are those of the opportunistic infections that take advantage of the damaged immune system. Many of the diseases are caused by fungi or viruses. This is because the T4 lymphocytes destroyed by HIV virus control cell-mediated immunity. It is this kind of immunity rather than the humoral immunity (see discussion on immune system in the previous chapter) that is mainly responsible for the body's defence against fungal, protozoal and viral infections.

The World Health Organization produced a clinical case definition for Africa (called the 'Bangui' case definition). This is also used outside Africa but some countries have replaced it with locally specific case definitions. The Bangui case definition is divided into the major and minor symptoms/signs as shown below. AIDS in an adult is defined by the existence of at least two of the major signs together with at least one minor sign in the absence of known causes of immunosuppression. The term AIDS-related illness can be used when the patient has some of the signs/symptoms and is HIV antibody positive but does not meet the full case definition.

The diagnostic diseases Kaposi's sarcoma or cryptococcal meningitis are sufficient by themselves for a diagnosis of AIDS.

Major signs

Chronic diarrhoea leading to a significant loss in weight is the most striking feature of AIDS. This led to the disease being called 'Slim' in Uganda. This is often accompanied by persistent fever and night sweats.

Minor signs

Enlarged lymph glands

The lymph nodes or glands are an important part of the body's immune system and are located in various parts of the body such as under the jaw, neck, armpits and groin. An early sign of AIDS is often painless bumps or swellings of at least one centimetre diameter in these lymph nodes. This is called 'persistent generalised lymphadenopathy' or PGL. Lymph node enlargement can also occur in other diseases such as glandular fever and tuberculosis.

Oropharyngeal candidiasis (oral thrush)

A common symptom of AIDS is a white furry coating on the tongue and roof of the mouth and sometimes the vagina. This is caused by a yeast *Candida albicans*. Candidiasis is not usually seen in healthy people because their immune systems are able to resist the infection. It can be seen in bottle-fed, ill babies and in debilitated elderly persons. In persons with a damaged immune system such as AIDS patients, candidiasis can persist for a long time and spread from the mouth to the gullet and lungs.

Chronic herpes simplex
Herpes simplex is a virus that produces sores – often called cold sores – in and around the mouth or in the genital or rectal areas. In people with a normal functioning immune system these sores are usually few in number, small in size and last only 2–3 days. In AIDS patients the sores are more severe and recur more often.

Recurrent herpes zoster (shingles)
When a child has chickenpox the virus stays in the body. It can become reactivated later in life and symptoms appear as an extremely painful rash. But shingles differs from chickenpox in that it is usually on only one side of the body. It usually appears on the trunk or face and stops exactly at the midline of the body. In the past shingles was an infection common in older people; now it has become a common opportunistic infection in younger people infected with HIV.

Pneumocystis carinii *pneumonia*
This is common in AIDS patients from America and Europe. It is caused by a microorganism (a protozoon) that infects the lungs and results in a form of pneumonia. It appears as a persistent dry cough; as the infection spreads the patient could develop a fatal pneumonia.

Diagnostic diseases

Kaposi's sarcoma
This is a cancer-like growth of the blood vessels which was very rare before 1980. It appears as dark raised areas on the skin that often first appear on the trunk or upper body and on the ears and nose. These skin nodules are not itchy or painful. The cancer can spread to internal organs and eventually cause death.

Cryptococcal meningitis
This is caused by a yeast-like fungus. Early symptoms include fever and mild headache followed by nausea, vomiting, headache and blurred vision. If untreated this disease is fatal.

Other symptoms found in AIDS patients

Tuberculosis (TB)
TB is another disease that can take advantage of a weakened immune system and develop in a patient. The symptoms are a persistent cough,

weight loss and coughing up blood. In many developing countries TB is the most common opportunistic infection associated with AIDS. It is also a very important cause of death in people with AIDS. Many countries are experiencing a substantial increase in TB because of AIDS.

Probably in most instances, tuberculosis infection is acquired before HIV. About 30–50% of adults in most developing countries have latent tuberculosis infection which can be demonstrated through a skin test. HIV-induced immunodeficiency is the strongest known risk factor for reactivation of latent tuberculosis.

AIDS dementia complex
The HIV virus can pass the blood-brain barrier and damage the brain, spinal cord and nerves. The effect will depend on the part of the brain affected. Symptoms could be strange unusual behaviour and confusion. Other symptoms could be paralysis or uncoordinated movements.

AIDS in children

HIV infection in children occurs mainly through two routes. Firstly, as explained in an earlier section, an HIV infected woman can pass on the infection to her unborn baby either before birth or at the time of birth. It has been estimated that between 15 and 35% of babies born to HIV antibody positive women are infected and will develop AIDS. Most of these children die by the age of 5 years.

As the graph of distribution of AIDS cases with age (Figure 5) shows, most children with AIDS are under 5 years of age and are infected from their mothers. The other group of children who have been found to have HIV infection are those who receive repeated transfusions of blood or blood products for blood disorders such as haemophilia or thalassaemia. In addition to these routes, an older adolescent child may become infected with HIV through sexual intercourse.

Some babies will have become infected through breast milk and this is discussed in the next chapter. A baby will carry his or her mother's antibodies for the first 12–18 months of life. An HIV antibody test during this period will not indicate whether a baby is infected with HIV, as a positive result might be due to the mother's antibodies.

The transition from being infected with HIV to the development of clinical AIDS and risk of repeated, severe infections, is quicker with babies than adults. However, there is considerable variation with some HIV positive infants dying in the first year of life and others surviving for more than 5 years. The clinical features in children are similar to those in adults, but the key features are growth faltering and repeated and severe infections, especially diarrhoea, pneumonia and fungal infections. Many of these features, however, also occur in babies with depressed immunity for other reasons – such as low birthweight or severe malnutrition. One cannot assume that a severely ill child is necessarily HIV positive.

WHO has adopted a provisional case definition where a child is considered to have AIDS when it has two of the major signs and two of the minor signs (herpes is not included among the minor signs), however this is not particularly satisfactory. It should be remembered that most HIV tests in developing countries use the ELISA which picks up antibodies against HIV. These can be transmitted from the mother to the infant and are detectable for 12–15 months after birth. The only way to be certain as to whether a baby is really infected with HIV is to perform the expensive polymerase chain reaction test that was discussed in the previous chapter.

Some vaccines used in immunisation contain live organisms that have been weakened so that they do not cause disease in a normal person. Some people have expressed concern whether it is advisable to give those immunisations to a child with HIV infection or AIDS. WHO has recommended that all children should continue to receive the full range of normal childhood immunisations including diphtheria, polio, tetanus, measles and mumps. WHO also recommends that BCG should be given to all children except when they show symptoms of HIV-related illnesses.

Treatment and outcome

There are three dimensions to management of patients with HIV/AIDS. Treating the underlying HIV infection, treating opportunistic infections and palliative/terminal care for persons at an advanced stage of AIDS. For detailed information on specific treatment regimes and drugs you should consult your National AIDS Programme, manufacturers instructions and the sources of information provided at the end of this book. UNAIDS provide a valuable technical update on treatment of HIV-related opportunistic diseases from which many of the specific treatment regimes below are drawn. Their excellent AIDS Home Care Manual provides a useful review of general care and support that can be provided by families and volunteers.

It is important to treat all medicines with respect. You should read the instructions carefully concerning when the medicines are to be taken, the size of dose appropriate to the patient's age and weight, and if there are particular groups that should not be given the medicine, e.g. children, pregnant women or persons on other medications. Many of the medicines named below should only be dispensed by trained health workers in situations where the patient can be followed up and medications changed if there are side effects. Some medicines can have side effects when given to persons with HIV/AIDS. These include sulfonamides and steroids. Steroids such as cortisone and hydrocortisone weaken the immune system and can worsen even further the situation of persons with HIV/AIDS.

For all the treatments described below, patients and their families should be given clear instructions on the use of any medicines that they are prescribed, possible side effects and the need for follow-up. These instructions should be supported wherever possible by written instructions using pictures and simple language.

Treatment of HIV infection

This involves slowing down the spread of the virus or removing it from the body (called decreasing the 'viral load'). Antibiotics work in this way in treating infections by bacteria, fungi and protozoa. However, antibiotics have not been found for *any* viral disease – not just for AIDS. It is also particularly difficult to treat AIDS because the virus hides itself in the genes of the cells it infects. HIV also destroys the immune system. Infection of brain cells by HIV and resulting AIDS dementia has already been described above. A drug would have to cross the blood-brain barrier to be effective.

The drugs that have been developed so far work in two different ways. The first group consists of the **reverse transcriptase inhibitors** which block the enzyme that is essential for HIV inserting itself into the infected person's genes. One class of reverse trancriptase inhibitors are named according to their chemical structure nucleoside analogues – examples of which include zidovudine (also called AZT), didanosine (ddI), zalcitabine (ddC) and lamivudine (3TC). Another class is the non-nucleoside analogues – an example of which is nevirapine.

The second group of drugs consists of the **protease inhibitors** and includes saquinavir, indinavir and ritonavir. These work by preventing the function of an enzyme that is essential for the formation of the different proteins that are needed to make up HIV in the human cell.

The third group of drugs that is being looked for, contains those drugs which might restore the damaged immune system of persons with HIV so that they can resist opportunistic infections.

The first treatment to be explored was AZT in the 1980s. This drug was found to have only a short-term effect on HIV which became resistant to its effect. However, a breakthrough was achieved in 1995 when trials showed that the use of two drugs together (combination therapy) had more impact that one alone. Since then there has been continued experimentation with different combinations with simultaneous use of up to four drugs and there is a general feeling of optimism about the future of persons with AIDS.

However, despite this optimism there are formidable problems to be overcome if the potential benefits of combination therapy are to be brought to the millions of people in the poor countries of the developing world where the need is greatest.

The drugs have to be taken for the rest of the infected persons life. The drugs are expensive – three drugs in combination can cost US$8,000 to US$20,000 a year. Taking the drugs involves following a complex schedule according to the time of day and with and without food. We already have the example of TB to show us how difficult it can be for poor people to follow long complicated programmes of treatment. If people do not take the drugs properly there is a real possibility of the spread of drug-resistant forms of HIV. Another problem is that most of the research on the use of combination therapy has been done with HIV1 and it is still unclear what are the best treatment approaches for infections with HIV2.

Some people experience side effects such as vomiting, diarrhoea, fever and diabetes. The drugs can interfere with other drugs the person may be taking.

Treatment is only possible when the drugs are available and there are health workers with the time and training to supervise their use and monitor the patients afterwards. Patient education has to be provided to carefully explain when and how to take the drugs, the side effects that may arise and the need to adopt safer sex practices including the use of condoms to protect their sexual partners. Follow-up is needed to ensure that drugs are having an impact on the patient's immune system (which will require taking blood samples for laboratory tests), to check for side effects and to prescribe alternative combinations of drugs if needed. At present many countries are examining their health policies to decide if they can afford to include drugs for treatment of HIV and resulting opportunistic infections within their essential drugs list and, if so, how much to charge for them. Difficult social, economic and ethical issues have to be resolved to ensure that access to combination therapy is not discriminated against by geography, gender, race, colour, religion or the ability to pay.

Treatment of opportunistic diseases

Treatment of opportunistic diseases – especially TB – can improve the AIDS patient's quality of life and prolong life. However these are only temporary solutions as the underlying cause, HIV infection, persists. With the lack of a functioning immune system the person will develop further opportunistic infections and eventually die. The distribution of symptoms and the availability and suitability of drugs vary between country and regions. Brief summaries are given below of some of the common and treatable opportunistic diseases in developing countries.

Tuberculosis

As described above TB is commonly found as a consequence of HIV infection and can be treated. Treatment of TB involves following a regime of drugs over a period of at least a year and a common problem has been is that patients may not complete their course of treatment. This can result in both renewed illness as well as antibiotic resistance. The DOTS ('Directly Observed Treatment Shortcourse') strategy involves use of combinations of antibiotics such as rifampicin, pyrazinamide, isoniazid, streptomycin and ethambutol that can be taken over a shorter time such as 6–8 months and needs intensive supervision of the patient either at the clinic by the health worker or in the home by volunteers to ensure that they complete their course. The anti-tuberculosis medicine, thioacetazone (also called 'thiazina') should not be given to persons with HIV/AIDS because it can lead to side effects. Effective patient education should explain both the need for full compliance and also the need for simple measures that the person with TB should take to prevent the infection of others such as covering his or her mouth when coughing and avoiding poorly ventilated areas. The DOTS procedure involves the following steps:

- diagnosis of TB by examination of sputum under a microscope and showing presence of bacilli (sputum test);
- providing a combination of drugs and clear advice on how and when they are used;
- observation of patients by volunteers and health workers and confirming that the drug doses have been followed;
- monitoring of treatment with a second sputum test after 2 months and at the end of treatment.

The DOTS process can produce cure rates of up to 95% even in the poorest countries. A 6 months supply of the drugs for DOTS costs US$11 per patient. The World Bank has described the DOTS strategy as one of the most 'cost effective of all health interventions'.

A recent breakthough was the discovery that giving antibiotics to HIV positive persons can reduce the likelihood of them going on to develop TB. This preventive therapy using isoniazid can be given to everyone who is found to be HIV positive. However, it is better to use a more selective approach and provide it to those persons who are carrying TB infection (as shown by a skin test) or those who live in areas where there are high levels of TB or in contact with TB patients. Before starting preventive therapy it is important to ensure that they do not already have clinical TB. If they have clinical TB they will need the full DOTS multi-drug treatment described above.

Fungal infections

The infections by the *Candida* yeast that causes thrush in the mouth, throat and vagina are distressing but not life-threatening. Infections in the mouth and throat can be painful and cause difficulty in swallowing. For thrush in the mouth it is best to start with the simple home remedy of gently cleaning the mouth with a soft toothbrush and rinsing the mouth with salt water (half a teaspoon in a cup of water) or lemon juice and then painting the infected surface three or four times a day with a solution of one teaspoon of gentian violet in half a litre of water. Localized infections in the mouth, throat and vagina can be treated by surface applications of anti-fungal agents such as nystatin, miconazole or clotrimazole. However, the yeast infection may be deeper and require treatment with systemic anti-fungal agents such as itraconazole, fluconazole or amphotericin B. Another common fungal infection, cryptococcal meningitis, is more difficult to treat and the drugs required are expensive and not readily available.

A very recent development is that when the drug co-trimoxazole is given to persons living with HIV/AIDS it can prevent the onset of *Pneumocystis carinii* pneumonia and some bacterial infections and prolong life.

Virus infections

Herpes simplex virus infection causes sores around the mouth and genitals and herpes zoster virus leads to localised rashes called shingles. These can both be extremely painful and in some cases can lead to life-threatening encephalitis. Herpes simplex can be treated with aciclovir, which only has a limited effect on herpes zoster. The itching from shingles can be reduced by applying calomine lotion twice daily and taking pain relief – see below. You can prevent infection by bathing sores in solutions of salt or gentian violet or application of antibiotic relief.

Weight loss and diarrhoea

Weight loss is one of the most dramatic signs of AIDS and can have many causes: tuberculosis, lack of absorption of nutrients because of diarrhoea and vomiting, difficulty in swallowing because of infections in the mouth and throat, problems in health of teeth and gums and a general loss of appetite and nausea as a consequence of various AIDS-related infections and psychosocial problems such as depression and anxiety.

A sick person has an even greater need for food than a healthy one, and it is important to encourage persons with AIDS to increase their intake of food. Some practical ways if increasing a sick person's food intake is to give them foods they enjoy, make the food soft and easily digestible and prepare smaller quantities but serve them more often. Foods such as groundnuts, when mashed and included in a meal, provide a simple way of providing more energy. It is also important to encourage a varied diet that includes fruit and vegetables.

The most important action to take when a person has diarrhoea is to drink plenty of fluids such as water, weak tea, fruit juice, soup, light porridge or rice water. It is important to continue feeding to prevent loss of weight and weakening (see above). Diarrhoea in infants and young children is especially serious as a small child can rapidly dehydrate to dangerous levels. Children under 2 years of age should be given a cup of water for each loose stool and continue to be fed. Breastfeeding mothers should continue to breastfeed a child with diarrhoea.

It is important to take prompt action if the diarrhoea continues and there are symptoms of dehydration such as feeling thirsty, irritable, tired, the skin going back slowly when pinched and – in the case of very young children – sunken eyes and fontanelle (the top of the skull). If there are signs of dehydration the person should be given oral rehydration solution. This can be obtained from health workers or pharmacists and made up by dissolving contents of an ORS packet in water in the correct amount of water (see instructions provided). Diarrhoea is the body's natural mechanism for removing harmful germs and toxins. Medicines such as co-phenotrope (Lomotil) which stop diarrhoea prevent this natural cleansing action and should be avoided.

Pain

Pain can be caused by HIV directly affecting the nerve fibres (peripheral neuropathy). Pain can also arise from opportunistic disease, general weakness, muscle ache and from bed sores from lying for too long in bed in one position. Pain can be experienced in the terminal stage of a disease when the patient is close to death. No-one should be allowed to suffer unnecessarily from pain. The approach to pain management recommended by WHO is initially to respond by giving simple painkillers such as aspirin and paracetamol which are available without prescription. Paracetamol can be harmful to the liver if the dose is exceeded and it is especially important when giving it to children to follow recommended doses. If these first-line treatments are not effective stronger painkillers can be used which should only be given under the supervision of trained health workers. This second-line treatment includes drugs such as codeine or dihydrocodeine, which could be combined with non-steroidal anti-inflammatory drugs such as ibuprofen or diclofenac. If these are not effective you can move the third level of morphine on its own or in combination with other painkillers. Some health workers avoid giving morphine to patients because they mistakenly believe that it might lead to drug addiction. However, when properly administered, addiction will not take place and the patient is spared considerable suffering.

Anxiety and depression

Anxiety may lead to symptoms such as lack of appetite, shaking, sweating, difficulty in sleeping, a feeling of being out of control and worried. Depression can result in a feeling of hopelessness, tiredness and lack of energy, inability to find pleasure, the sense that everything is a chore, inability to concentrate and poor memory, waking up early in the morning or having trouble getting to sleep at night. Everyone experiences some of these symptoms at some stage in their life as a natural response to the demands of life. However, if the situation persists, it can prevent a person meeting the everyday demands of life, and can lead to people harming themselves or considering extreme measures such as suicide. Not surprisingly, the diagnosis of infection with HIV/AIDS is a time of shock, crisis and stress for the patient and his/her family. The impact of this can to some extent be minimised with proper pre- and post-test counselling which are discussed more fully in Chapter 6. Counselling and appropriate home-care services should be the first line of treatment for depression. However, if this is not enough you can ask a health worker to prescribe medication.

Palliative and terminal care

Palliative care for persons with AIDS includes medical and nursing care, social and emotional support and counselling and spiritual needs. The aim is to maintain the quality of life of the person and develop a positive approach to their illness. The aim of terminal care is to provide the necessary support to enable a person to die with dignity. Both palliative and terminal care can include the treatment of opportunistic infections and management of pain discussed above combined with broader psychosocial aspects of counselling and home-based care which are discussed in Chapter 6.

Alternative and traditional medicine

Alongside the developments in anti-viral therapy described above, there have been repeated and unsubstantiated claims of miracle cures from people who are prepared to make money out of people's desperate search for a cure. An example of the harm that can be done by premature and unproven claims of cures was the blaze of publicity following the launching on the 27th July 1990 of a drug Kemron in Kenya. More recently an apparent cure for AIDS was announced in South Africa for a substance called Virodene – with no evidence to support its claims for effectiveness.

Many countries have practitioners of 'non-western', 'traditional' or 'alternative' medicine. These are often highly respected and have their associations and training programmes. Some traditional healers have claimed to have found cures for AIDS and successfully treated persons. These claims have been given widespread publicity in the press. The public is desperate for news of a miracle cure and will readily believe false claims. Often what the traditional healers have been doing is treating the opportunistic infections. This may make the person feel better for a while but not deal with the underlying problem of the damaged immune system. In other cases of apparent cure it may have been that the original diagnosis was wrong and that the person did not have AIDS.

Traditional healers are a valuable resource in the community and provide much comfort and care. With suitable training and support, they have a major role to play in psychosocial aspects of care, the treatment of opportunistic infections and referral of persons with sexually transmitted diseases. You should spend time explaining to them about AIDS and sexually transmitted diseases and involving them in your programmes. You should keep an open mind about the possibility of a cure for AIDS being discovered by a traditional healer. But any cure, either from western or non-western medicine, should be properly tested to make sure it is both safe and effective and does not raise false hopes.

Concluding remarks on treatment

This chapter has provided background information on the symptoms and treatment of persons with HIV and AIDS. More information will be provided in Chapter 6 on how this information can be integrated into counselling and community-based care. With the developments in combination therapy in recent years, it is possible to take a more optimistic view than previous editions of this book. Hopefully there will be more progress in future in the development of simple, affordable and accessible treatment for HIV. Increasing globalisation of multi-national drug companies put them outside the control of individual governments. A sustained effort by the international community is needed to ensure that the search for more profits by drug companies is not at the expense of the poor. In the absence of progress we must continue to look to prevention as the main strategy for the control of AIDS. The next chapter will review our knowledge about the way the virus is transmitted from person to person and how this information can be used for the prevention of AIDS.

4. Transmission

HIV is present in all body fluids of an infected person but is concentrated in blood, semen and vaginal fluids. It is present in virtually all body tissues and organs including the brain, spinal cord, cerebrospinal fluid and breast milk. It can be found in tears and saliva although these are not considered significant routes of infection.

Many people are afraid of HIV and AIDS. However, the good news is that it does not spread from person to person very easily. Viruses such as those of the common cold or influenza are tough viruses that are able to withstand buffeting in air and are highly infectious. HIV is a delicate virus that is easily killed by heat and by drying. A larger dose of virus is needed to spread HIV than another virus that is spread in a similar way, hepatitis B. Four critical conditions must be fulfilled if HIV is to be transmitted by a particular route:

- HIV must be present in a body fluid. In practice this means semen, vaginal fluids, blood or blood products.
- HIV must survive during the period it is out of the body. This can be a long time in stored blood but is quite short in most other situations.
- HIV must get into a person. Skin forms a barrier to HIV so the virus must enter where the skin is damaged or more delicate, e.g. the mucous membranes of the anus and vagina. The acid in the stomach inactivates the virus.
- Sufficient HIV must be transferred into the other person to make an infective dose.

Sexual transmission

The main route for the spread of HIV is by sexual intercourse between two people when one person is carrying the virus. Vaginal intercourse, where the penis of the male penetrates the vagina of the female is a common route of transmission. Anal intercourse, where the penis penetrates the anus of the other person, can also be a route of transmission. Semen is a mixture of sperm and seminal fluid. HIV is not in sperm. However, it is present as free virus particles in seminal fluid and also within cells from the immune system which are also present in semen. Artificial insemination, where semen from a man is artificially inserted into a female could also be a route of infection. An HIV antibody positive man who has had a vasectomy could still infect another person because the seminal fluid will still contain HIV.

A single sexual encounter can be sufficient to transmit HIV. However some studies suggest that the risk from a single act of intercourse between a male and female can be as low as one chance in one thousand.

However, the likelihood of HIV being transmitted during sexual intercourse can be much greater. Although the risk from an individual sexual act may be low, the more times a person has sex, the greater the likelihood that transmission will take place. Women appear to be more at risk than men from heterosexual sex. The transmission of HIV from man to woman is believed to take place more easily than woman to man. This is not an easy area to research as it is necessary to study couples where one partner is known to be infected with HIV and the other is not (discordant couples). In their Draft Global Strategic Plan for Women and AIDS produced in 1993, WHO estimated that male-to-female transmission could be two to four times more efficient than female-to-male. The most likely reason is that the semen from the man remains in the woman for a period of time and thus increases the likelihood of transmission. Another reason is that the vagina can be damaged during intercourse. This is especially likely with a young woman and the risk of transmission through sex is considered to be particularly high for teenage girls. Female circumcision (also called female genital mutilation) is practised in some communities and the damage to the female genital area is also likely to increase the risk of transmission.

The risk of HIV infection will also depend on how much virus the person has in their body. That will depend on the stage in the disease and whether the person is receiving combination therapy.

Other ways in which the efficiency of sexual intercourse in transmission of HIV is increased are described below.

Sexually transmitted diseases

Any sores on the penis or the walls of the vagina can increase the chance of HIV transmission. One common reason for this is the presence of a sexually transmitted disease such as syphilis or chancroid. Sexually transmitted diseases (STDs) – also called sexually transmitted infections (STIs) – is a general term which includes sexually transmitted infections and all the complications including infertility that might follow. These diseases cause sores or genital ulcers in and around the sexual organs. These provide breaks in the skin through which HIV can pass.

Another reason for the effect of sexually transmitted diseases on HIV transmission is that the pus or exudate from sores on the genital areas and discharges from the penis are rich in white blood cells. As stated above, semen contains also contains cells from the immune system. In an infected person, this pus and semen will contain HIV and increase the risk of transmission to the sexual partner.

In the traditional approach, sexually transmitted diseases were grouped according to the specific disease, e.g. gonorrhoea, syphilis etc. There is increasing interest in the *syndromic approach* using the four categories of symptoms in the box:

Sexually Transmitted Diseases (syndromic approach)

Vaginal discharge (women):
Abnormal discharges from the vagina are a sign of a STD. They can be white, brown, yellow or milky with or without offensive odour. They may be accompanied by itching, a burning sensation or pain when passing urine or during sexual intercourse.

Vaginal discharges can be caused by: gonorrhoea, chlamydia, candidiasis, trichomoniasis and bacterial vaginosis. These abnormal discharges result from the damage the infection is causing to the reproductive organs. If left untreated, these STDs can lead to: infertility, abnormal pregnancies, miscarriages, stillbirths, abnormalities/eye discharges in new-born babies.

Genital ulcers (men and women)
Genital ulcers are sores on the surface and inside the male or female sex organs. There could be one or more ulcers, smooth or ragged, clean or full of pus, painful or painless and they may be accompanied by lumps in the lymph nodes in the groin.

The STDs that cause them are: syphilis, genital herpes, lymphogranuloma venereum, chancroid, granuloma inguinale. The ulcers result from damage to the skin by germs. If untreated this can lead to complications such as damage to the genital organs, delivery of abnormal babies and sometimes brain damage. Genital ulcers are very serious and can greatly increase the risk of acquiring HIV.

Urethral discharge (men)
A discharge from the penis is the most common symptom of STDs for men. It is caused by an infection of the urine passage. The discharge appears 2–21 days after infection. The nature of the discharge depends on the specific disease. It could be milky, yellowish, brownish, green or blood-stained in colour.

It could be as a result of any of the following infections: gonorrhoea, chlamydia, genital herpes and non-specific urethritis. If the infection is not treated, it can lead to blockage of the urinary passage, damage to the testicles and infertility.

> **Lower abdominal pain (women)**
> This can be caused by pelvic inflammatory disease and be a result of infection with sexually transmitted diseases such as gonorrhoea and chlamydia. However, other factors that are not STDs can also cause this including complications of pregnancy, abortion, intestinal obstruction and appendicitis so a careful examination is needed before a STD is diagnosed.

Menstruation

A woman with HIV will have the virus in her menstrual blood. Sexual intercourse during her periods will be more risky than out of menstruation. Her sanitary pads or tampons will also contain HIV.

Anal intercourse

Anal sex is the name for sexual intercourse where the penis is inserted into the other person's anus. It is common among male homosexuals but is also practised among heterosexuals. It is of particularly high risk for the transmission of HIV and this is because the wall of the lining of the anus is delicate and is easily torn when the penis is inserted. Also there are many white blood cells in the blood vessels feeding the rectum. These cells will become infected when they come into contact with semen containing HIV. If a person is HIV antibody positive the white blood cells in the rectal blood vessels will be rich in virus particles. Any bleeding during intercourse will lead to infected blood coming into contact with the penis of the sex partner.

Homosexuality

Homosexuals are persons who prefer to have sex with persons of their own sex. The term 'gay' is often used to describe male–male relationships and 'lesbian' is used for female–female relationships. A bisexual is a person who has both heterosexual and homosexual sex.

The AIDS epidemics in USA and Europe were initially among male homosexuals and only later began to spread among the heterosexual population. This contrasts with the situation in Africa and the Caribbean where the main way HIV has been transmitted is through heterosexual intercourse.

The coming of AIDS has led to a greater willingness to talk about homosexuality. It is now generally accepted that homosexuality is more widespread than had been realised. In addition there are many persons who see themselves as heterosexual, are married and with children, but who occasionally have sex with men. Homosexual sex is also practised by heterosexuals away from their families in institutional settings such as prisons and hostels.

Unfortunately the AIDS epidemic has also led to an increase in prejudice against homosexuals or 'homophobia'. However, the reasons why AIDS has been so widespread among homosexuals has not been because of homosexuality itself. It was probably accidental that HIV became introduced to male homosexual groups in USA and Europe. These groups formed tight-knit communities where multiple partner sex and anal intercourse were common practices. This is possibly the reason for the rapid spread of HIV in this group (also called the 'gay' community). These early infected persons travelled to other parts of the USA and abroad where they spread it to other homosexual communities.

Female homosexual intercourse, or lesbianism, is considered a very low risk activity for transmission of HIV.

Masturbation

This involves the stimulation by hand of the sexual organs. This can be either self-masturbation when a person stimulates his or her own sexual organs or mutual masturbation between two partners. There is no risk of transmission of HIV from self-masturbation because only one person is involved. Provided semen or vaginal fluid from one person does not come into contact with the sex organs of the other, mutual masturbation is a very low risk activity. There may be a slight risk if the hand used to stimulate the other person's sexual organ has cuts or sores.

Blood routes

Blood transfusions

There is no risk of becoming infected with HIV by giving blood as the equipment used is normally sterile. However receiving blood contaminated with HIV will lead to infection. Many persons in the developed and developing countries have contracted HIV from blood transfusions. For example, in Zaire a study found that HIV positive adults and children were twice as likely to have had a blood transfusion as people who were not infected.

Common reasons for blood transfusions are anaemias from thalassaemia, sickle-cell anaemia and malaria. Women, because of problems of anaemia and childbirth complications, tend to receive more blood transfusions than men. Although widespread screening of blood has virtually eliminated blood as a source of HIV infection in USA and Europe, this is still not the case in many developing countries.

Since late 1985 most western countries have been testing blood for HIV and this practice is increasingly being adopted in developing countries. Unfortunately contaminated blood is still a route of infection for HIV in some developing countries where difficulties have been encountered in setting up safe blood transfusion systems. Even when systems for testing are in place, these need continual monitoring to ensure that they are effective. In Germany a scandal erupted in 1993 when it was realised that a private company, UB Plasma, was selling blood products to hospitals throughout Germany and other countries without properly testing them for HIV. Some doctors believe that up to 1000 persons have been infected and the factory has been closed down.

The testing of blood does not remove all risk from transmission through donated blood. It takes 3–12 weeks after infection for the body to produce antibodies. If blood is donated during this 'window' period antibodies will not be detected by the HIV test but the blood will still be infectious. It is therefore important that blood transfusions are given only when necessary.

Haemophiliacs and Factor 8

Haemophiliacs have a genetic deficiency that prevents their blood from clotting in cases of cuts and injuries. They require regular supplies of a substance called Factor 8 that is made from blood. Many haemophiliacs in USA and Europe were infected with HIV through receiving Factor 8 made from contaminated blood. All blood used to make Factor 8 is now heat-treated to destroy the HIV virus.

Injecting drug users

Another way by which contaminated blood can be passed from person to person is through injecting drugs. The main drug injected worldwide is heroin, followed by cocaine and amphetamines. When people inject drugs such as heroin they frequently draw in a small amount of blood into the syringe. If someone else uses the same needle that blood containing the HIV virus will be injected and lead to infection. Injecting drug users form tight-knit communities. Once HIV infects one person it can spread rapidly throughout the network of drug injectors.

In South-East Asia – especially Thailand, Myanmar, India and Yunnan Province in China – injection by drug abusers is emerging as an important route of infection. In Myanmar, a dramatic increase in HIV seropositivity has been documented among injecting drug users from 17% in 1989 to 59% and 71% in 1990 and 1991 respectively. In

1991 the National Institute of Cholera and Enteric Diseases (NICED) in India found 80% of 273 intravenous drug users in a town in Manipur, North India, to be infected with HIV.

Injecting drugs is increasing in many countries and becoming a worldwide phenomenon. In Africa drug injection was once considered rare but is increasingly being reported.

Once drug injectors are infected with HIV, they can also transmit the virus to others through sexual intercourse or, when pregnant, to their babies. Many injecting drug users also act as sex workers to pay for their drugs and this was a significant factor in the rapid early spread of AIDS in Thailand.

Injections

A possible route of infection for HIV (and other diseases such as hepatitis B and C) is through injections by health workers when needles and syringes have not been properly sterilised. There have been occasions when there have been shortages of needles and well intentioned health workers have reused them without sterilisation. It is not clear how important this route of infection has been in developing countries and early fears that HIV was being spread through immunization programmes were probably exaggerated. However there have been studies in Zaire, Rwanda and Haiti that found that HIV positive people had received more injections 1–5 years previously than healthy persons. The transmission of HIV to children through contaminated injections has also been reported in the former Soviet Union and Romania. A recent review supported by the World Health Organization estimates that unsafe injection practices lead to 80–160 thousand deaths from HIV/AIDS each year. If the other diseases such as hepatitis B and C are also considered, the total global burden from unsafe injection practices amounts to 1.3 million deaths each year.

All injections can transmit HIV. However, injections into veins (intravenous injections) appear to be much more likely to spread HIV than intradermal, subcutaneous or intramuscular injections.

In some developing countries there are persons with little health-care training who have set themselves up as private practitioners and give injections. If these syringes are not properly sterilised, there is a risk of spread of HIV.

Other practices involving skin piercing

The risks to health workers through needlestick injuries and cuts is discussed later in this chapter.

There are a variety of practices that involve piercing the skin with instruments which, if they are not sterilised, might lead to transmission of HIV. Examples of this in Europe, USA and Asia are acupuncture and tattooing. Controls have been introduced in many countries to ensure that the instruments used are sterilised properly.

In Africa there are some traditional practices involving skin piercing. These include circumcision, facial markings, and healing practices involving placing of herbs in cuts in the skin. In Asia tattooing, ear/nose piercing and circumcision are common skin piercing practices. There is no evidence that these traditional practices have played a significant part in the spread of AIDS in Africa or Asia.

Practices that are part of a community's heritage and culture should be respected. However, it is important that they are carried out such a way that they do not lead to HIV transmission. Efforts should be made to ensure that they are carried out with sterilised instruments.

Circumcision

Male circumcision is practised in many cultures and involves cutting off the foreskin on the penis. This is often done on babies but in many cultures it is carried out as a traditional ceremony when a group of boys are circumcised together.

There is evidence from some studies that a circumcised male is less likely to acquire sexually transmitted diseases and HIV from sexual intercourse. This is because in the uncircumcised male, vaginal secretions from an infected female sex partner containing HIV and other STD causing germs may be retained within the foreskin after sexual intercourse. The foreskin can also become damaged during intercourse allowing HIV to enter through breaks in the skin.

The above beneficial effects may be offset by risks from circumcision. Although it has not been demonstrated, it is theoretically possible that HIV might be transferred from person to person if the same knife is used without sterilisation between persons. However, as it is often young boys who are circumcised in group ceremonies, they are less likely to have HIV and the risk is probably small.

Female circumcision, also called female genital mutilation, is practised by some societies in Africa and the Middle East. This dangerous practice involves removing part of the clitoris and other sexual organs. This might involve some risk of infection if the blade is not sterilised. The effect of this practice is a restriction of the vaginal area that can lead to damage and tearing during intercourse. This damage is likely to increase the risk of HIV transmission during sexual intercourse.

Tissue and organ transplants

Any exchange of infected tissue such as skin grafts and organ transplants could provide a mechanism for transmission of HIV from an infected donor. There is no evidence that this has played an important role in the past but it needs to be included in advice for HIV antibody positive persons.

Mother-to-child transmission

The likelihood that a mother who is HIV antibody positive will give birth to an infected baby is 15–25% for a mother who does not breastfeed and 25–45% for a mother who breastfeeds. The mechanism by which infection is passed on to children is a subject of intense research in order to find ways in which it could be reduced. This is not an easy area for research because all babies born to HIV infected mothers will test positive for HIV because of the antibodies they have received from their mother. Only after waiting a few months or carrying out expensive antigen tests is it possible to find out whether a baby is infected.

A baby can become infected in three ways:

1. HIV can cross the placenta from the mother to the infant before birth – especially during the last three months of pregnancy. The risk of infection depends on how much virus is in the mother. A mother with AIDS is more likely to give birth to an infected baby than a mother who is infected by HIV but has not yet developed symptoms. Risk of transmission through the placenta is increased when the mother has become infected with HIV during pregnancy.
2. HIV can also be transmitted from the mother when the baby travels down the birth canal during birth. A drawn out labour and a long time between rupture of the membranes and delivery are believed to increase risk of transmission. Delivery by Caesarian section before rupture of the membranes will reduce the risk of HIV transmission.
3. Some transmission also takes place through breastfeeding (see below).

UNAIDS has estimated that for every 100 breast-fed infants that were infected by their mothers: 20 will have been infected during pregnancy, 45–50 during delivery and 30–35 through breastfeeding.

Breastfeeding

Recent research has sadly confirmed that breastfeeding is a major route by which HIV can be passed on from an infected mother to her child. The evidence for this has come from study of babies when the mother had become infected after birth through a blood transfusion or sexual intercourse. The higher rate of transmission from mothers to children in developing than developed countries can now be explained by the fact that more mothers breastfeed.

HIV has been found in both colostrum and breast milk of HIV-infected mothers. The risk of transmission through breast milk is likely to increase according to how long the baby is breast-fed, whether the mother has sores or cracked nipples and if the mother becomes infected while breastfeeding.

Oral routes of infection

Saliva, ingestion through the mouth and kissing

HIV has been detected in saliva (and most other body fluids) and this has raised worries about the possibility of catching AIDS through kissing or sharing utensils. The concentration of virus in saliva, however, is very low and there are substances in saliva that can inactivate HIV. Even if virus is swallowed the acid in the stomach would inactivate HIV. There may be a slight risk from deep kissing where the tongues of the persons penetrate each other's mouths. Infection through kissing might take place when one partner has cuts or sores in the mouth that provide a point of entry for the virus. There is no risk from kissing on the cheek.

The low risk from saliva is supported by a study carried out in Canada of 30 health workers who had received bites from a patient who had AIDS and was mentally disturbed. Even after 2½ years, none of them became infected with HIV.

Mouth-to-mouth resuscitation

First-aid workers have been worried about the risk of giving mouth-to-mouth resuscitation to people with HIV. In most situations the risk is similar to kissing and very low. There may be a very small risk when the patient is bleeding from the mouth. The International Red Cross and Crescent Society recommends that first-aid workers should wipe off any blood from the injured person's mouth when doing mouth-to-mouth resuscitation. Plastic one-way valves are also available for resuscitation.

Oral sex

Oral sex can be done in different ways. The tongue of one partner can contact and stimulate the penis or vagina of the other partner. Semen or vaginal fluid can enter the mouth of the partner. Saliva can come into contact with the genitals of the other partner.

Oral sex carries greater risk of transmission of HIV than kissing for the person who is receiving the semen in his or her mouth. Sucking the genitals of a person with HIV can lead to a larger quantity of HIV entering the mouth than would take place during kissing. This might lead to infection if there are cuts or sores in the mouth. In the year 2000, the Centers for Disease Control and University of California reported on a study of 102 gay and bi-sexual men which found that eight of the men had been infected through oral sex. Although the risk is low, it is clearly significant and oral sex cannot be recommended as a safer-sex alternative to other methods of sexual intercourse.

Other routes by which HIV is not transmitted

Faeces and urine

Faeces and urine contain very little HIV. In some situations, such as dysentery or intestinal bleeding, there may be blood in the faeces and in this case there might be HIV in faeces. Even so, casual contact through handling these faeces is unlikely to lead to infection. Although faeces can transmit a wide range of other diseases, they are not a route of infection for HIV.

Transmission by insects

Many people worry that AIDS and HIV can be transmitted when insects such as mosquitoes and bed bugs draw blood from a person with HIV and then bite another.

There are three reasons why we know HIV is not transmitted by mosquitoes:

1. The amount of virus in the blood that the mosquito takes up is too small to enable reinfection. In malaria there is replication of the parasite in the mosquito that increases the infection dose but HIV is not able to replicate in mosquitoes.
2. If HIV was insect borne we would expect all age groups to be affected including children. As shown in graphs such as Figure 5, children between the ages of 3 and 14 rarely become infected by HIV but commonly suffer from malaria.
3. A pattern of insect transmission would result in all members of a family being exposed to HIV. Studies of AIDS and HIV in families

have shown that it is the sexual partner of the infected person who is at risk and not other members of the household.

Casual contact

The skin forms a natural barrier and HIV is not transmitted through any of the following ways (see also Figure 6):

- casual contact such as touching, shaking hands,
- from toilets, urinals, sharing towels, utensils, cups and saucers,
- from swimming pools and village ponds.

Fear of AIDS has led to unwillingness to work alongside persons with HIV or allow children with HIV to go to school. This can be very stressful to the HIV antibody positive person. This negative reaction is due to misconceptions about the transmission of HIV because there is very little risk of infection by HIV through normal contact.

Risks to health workers

Health workers frequently come into close contact with patients and their body fluids. Understandably many health workers worry that they may become infected with HIV.

Nurses and midwives are often in contact with blood. Laboratory workers handle blood samples, ward attendants and cleaners transport blood, faeces, sanitary towels, syringes and broken glass. There can be shortages of plastic gloves, protective aprons and proper disposal facilities. A common accident that can take place is when health workers accidentally prick themselves with syringes and other 'sharps'.

Health workers and ambulance drivers can be concerned from the risks attached to giving first aid such as mouth-to-mouth resuscitation.

Surgeons and nurses performing operations come into contact with blood and can accidentally cut themselves. Midwives come in contact with blood during childbirth. There are also traditional birth attendants who carry out many deliveries in rural communities with little training or support.

As described in earlier sections of this chapter, HIV is not transmitted through casual contact but through sexual intercourse and situations where blood products enter another person's bloodstream. The risk of catching HIV from contact with patients is believed to be very low for most health workers.

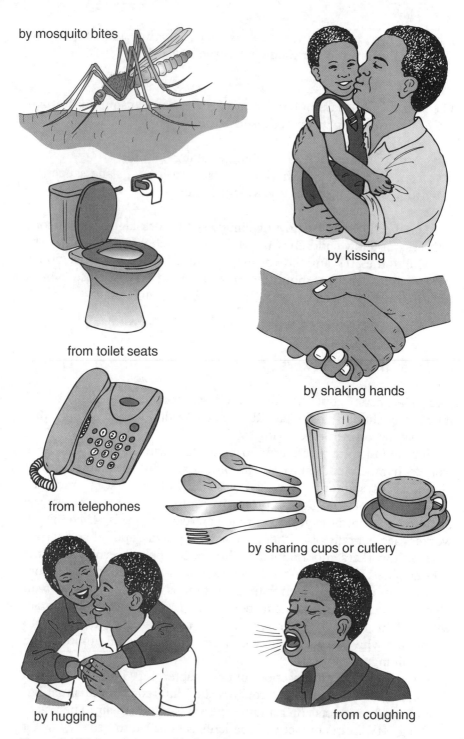

by mosquito bites

by kissing

from toilet seats

by shaking hands

from telephones

by sharing cups or cutlery

by hugging

from coughing

Figure 6. HIV does not spread in these ways

Some of the most detailed studies of risk to health workers have been carried out by the Centers for Disease Control (CDC) in United States. By mid 1998, there had been more than 600,000 reported cases of AIDS in the United States resulting in millions of hours of patient to health care worker contact. However, despite this, up to the end of June 1998, the CDC had recorded only 55 cases of health care workers who had definitely become infected from their health work. In addition there were a further 136 cases in which infection from health work was possible but not proven. These 55 included 19 laboratory workers, 23 nurses and six doctors. Most of these (47 out of the 54) were from needlestick injuries or cuts, five were a result of splashes of blood on skin and mucous membranes (eyes and inside of nose or mouth) and two were a combination of the two and one case of unknown origin. Some of these infections were due to improper disposal or re-capping of needles. Many of the exposures involved sharp objects penetrating through gloves.

For a needlestick accident to lead to HIV infection a sufficiently large quantity of infected blood must be injected into the health worker. The risk of infection by HIV from a needlestick injury has been estimated as one in three hundred (0.3%). This is much lower than the risk for transmission through needlestick injury of hepatitis C (6%) and hepatitis B (20–40%). The risk after exposure of the eye, nose or mouth to splashes of HIV-infected blood has been estimated as one in a thousand.

In a classic study of almost 2400 hospital workers in Zaire in 1988 the number of seropositive persons was no higher in the health workers who had contact with AIDS patients than the administrative staff and manual workers who did not have such contact. The seropositive persons in both groups were most likely infected through their personal lives rather than through working contact with patients.

The general conclusion from most researchers is that health workers are at low risk of catching HIV through contact with patients, provided the normal precautions of patient care are followed. These precautions are described in the next chapter.

Risk of transmission from health worker to patient

A report from the United States of the transmission of HIV from a dentist to five of his patients attracted a considerable publicity. In the United Kingdom there has been widespread concern by patients of doctors who later were discovered to be HIV antibody positive. However, the risk of transmission from health worker to patient through

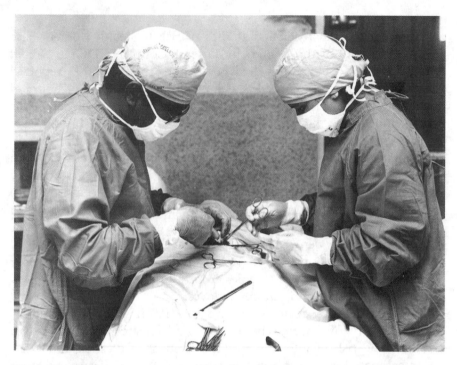

Figure 7. Health workers are at low risk of becoming infected with HIV if they follow normal hospital procedures

normal patient contact is extremely low. The Centers for Disease Control in United States studied 15,000 patients of 32 HIV-infected doctors and dentists and found no cases of HIV transmission from contact with the health workers.

Risk to families of AIDS patients

Family members and neighbours of HIV positive persons and AIDS patients are at virtually no risk of becoming infected with HIV through ordinary casual contact with the person or their clothing and utensils. However, the sexual partner of the infected person has a real risk of contracting HIV through sexual intercourse. Counselling on safer sexual practices should always be provided to the infected person and his/her sexual partner (see Chapter 6). Guidelines for family members who care for infected persons are given in the next two chapters.

5. Prevention of AIDS

Without accessible treatment we must look to prevention as our main hope for overcoming this fatal disease. This section will draw on the discussions of the routes of transmission in the previous chapter and will look at the various ways in which the transmission of HIV can be prevented.

Prospects for development of a vaccine

Vaccines have been successfully developed against many viral diseases such as polio, smallpox and measles. The development of a vaccine against HIV is an important objective for preventing the spread of infection.

Vaccines involve injecting solutions of fragments of the dead virus or a weakened non-lethal version of the live virus. This stimulates the body's immune defence system so that it can effectively resist future infections by HIV. In the attempt to find a vaccine for AIDS, three different kinds of vaccine are being explored. *Prophylactic* or preventive vaccines would prevent HIV from establishing itself in a person's body. *Therapeutic* or treatment vaccines would slow down or reverse the development of symptoms of AIDS in a person already infected with the virus. *Peri-natal vaccines* would prevent HIV infected women from passing the virus to their babies. So far the most likely prospect is for a prophylactic vaccine.

Developing a vaccine is not easy. If a fragment of the virus is used, careful attention must be given to choosing which fragment will perform best. A live virus must be chemically treated so that it is not capable of causing AIDS. A particular problem with HIV is that the virus can change its genetic composition and this changes the envelope of the virus. A vaccine developed from the envelope of one strain of the virus may not be effective against another type/sub-type of HIV.

The testing of a vaccine for effectiveness and safety is a long process. There are several trials of vaccines in progress. These have passed animal tests and the first phase of being tested on small groups of human volunteers and a second phase of tests with larger groups. A third phase of field trials among larger groups in the community has begun in USA and Thailand and hopefully further large scale trials will begin in other countries. Unfortunately, the vaccine that is at its most advanced stage of development has been developed against clades B of HIV-1. This is the subtype that is mainly found in developed countries Europe, North America and Australia. A vaccine that is effective against this type would not be as effective in preventing infection from sub-type A and C which are found mainly in developing countries.

In 1996 the International AIDS Vaccine Initiative (IAVI) was set up to promote the development of HIV vaccines. In 1997 President Clinton of the USA set a 10-year target for the development of an HIV vaccine – a goal which he considered equivalent to that set in 1961 by President Kennedy for putting a man on the moon. Sadly, even 2007 looks unlikely for a safe and effective vaccine.

Changes in sexual lifestyles

The most important way to prevent the spread of HIV is for people to ensure that their sexual behaviour does not put themselves at risk. Two major changes in sexual behaviour are needed: the *reduction in the number of sexual partners* and the *move from high-risk to low-risk sexual activities*.

Check list: Does your lifestyle put you at risk?

Some idea of your own risk of becoming infected with HIV can be obtained from the following questions. The more questions you answer YES the more at risk you are.

- Have you had more than one partner in the last year?
- Is there a chance that your partner is unfaithful to you?
- Do you have sex with sex workers (prostitutes)?
- Do you inject drugs such as heroin?
- Do you neglect to use condoms in sexual encounters with unfamiliar partners?

Reduction in the number of partners

Abstaining completely from sex is the safest way of avoiding infection but is unrealistic for most people! Even delaying sex until marriage is now becoming less common. Below are a range of activities ranging from no risk to high risk.

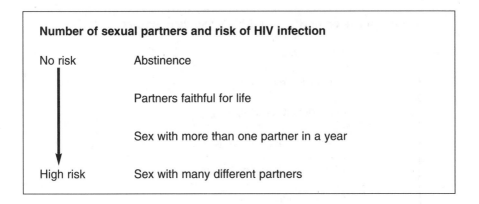

Number of sexual partners and risk of HIV infection

No risk   Abstinence

       Partners faithful for life

       Sex with more than one partner in a year

High risk   Sex with many different partners

Restricting the number of sex partners or delaying sex until marriage will not guarantee avoiding AIDS. You cannot tell from appearances whether your partner is carrying HIV. A person may have contracted the virus from a single sexual encounter more than 5 years ago and since then have had few sex partners. The most effective way of ensuring that your partner does not have HIV (and your partner will also want to be certain about you!) will be for each of you to have an antibody test for HIV. Many of the persons who come to the voluntary counselling and testing services in Uganda (described in the next chapter) are couples who are at the point of deciding whether to start a relationship or get married. Unfortunately, testing services are still not widely available in many countries.

The above approach assumes that both partners are prepared to discuss these sensitive issues together, delay sexual intercourse and modify their sexual practices. For many people the decision to have intercourse is one that is not made logically and reasoned out but governed by emotions and passion as well as family and community pressures. This issue of whether to have a test is one that requires careful thought. It may involve facing up to the discovery that you are HIV antibody positive.

Given these problems of determining the HIV status of one's sex partner, it is important to identify ways of continuing to have sex but reducing the chances of contracting HIV.

Low risk forms of sexual intercourse

As discussed in the section on transmission, not all types of sexual activities carry the same risk. The following box summarises the risks attached to different activities.

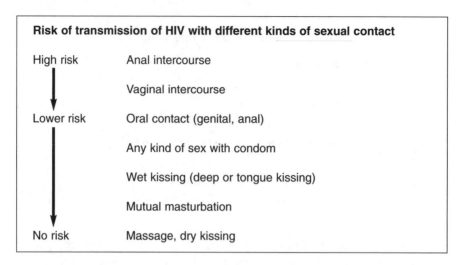

Risk of transmission of HIV with different kinds of sexual contact

High risk — Anal intercourse

Vaginal intercourse

Lower risk — Oral contact (genital, anal)

Any kind of sex with condom

Wet kissing (deep or tongue kissing)

Mutual masturbation

No risk — Massage, dry kissing

Condoms

A condom is a thin membrane tube usually made from latex rubber that covers the penis and prevents semen from entering the vagina (see Figure 8). Condoms can also be used for anal intercourse although stronger ones are recommended. Other names for condom are rubber, french letter, durex and even raincoats and gumboots!

Condoms have been available for a long time and have been promoted both as a method for family planning and for prevention of sexually-transmitted diseases. Condoms have a reputation for not being very reliable as a family planning method. However, many of these failures have been because the users had only just started using condoms. Among experienced users failure rates of as little as 0.4–2% have been found.

In many countries strict quality control and testing procedures for condoms are enforced. As a result, the actual risk from bursting is very low and usually less than 1% in newly-manufactured latex condoms. However, the risk of breakage can increase dramatically to more than 30% if the condoms are stored in very hot conditions, exposed to direct sunlight or crushed during stacking (or even in a back pocket!). People may not use condoms every time they have sex, condoms may be re-used or damaged during putting on. If care is not taken they can come off during withdrawal. The reasons for failure emphasise the importance of education for proper use (see guidelines below).

There is evidence from investigations in both laboratory and field situations that condoms can prevent the transmission of HIV and other STDs. Laboratory studies have shown that the HIV virus cannot pass through the thin membrane of the condom (even air and water do not pass through the condom and these molecules are much smaller than HIV). It is much more difficult, both for ethical and practical reasons, to set up experiments to prove the effectiveness of condoms in real life situations. In 1994 a multi-country European follow-up for

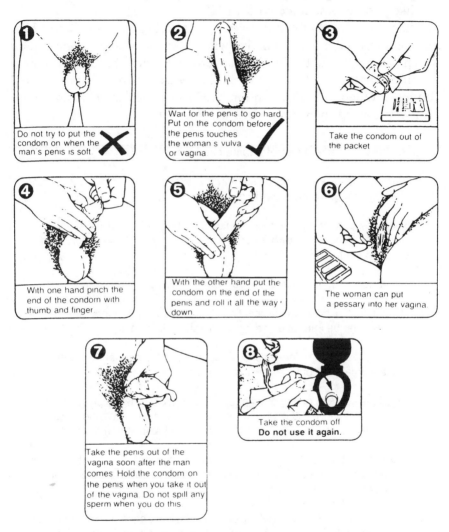

Figure 8. How to use a condom (illustrations taken from a leaflet produced by the Brook Advisory Centres)

20 months found not one case of HIV transmission among those couples who used condoms consistently each time. Evidence is also available from studies of female sex workers in Kenya and Zaire and other studies of HIV transmission that regular users of condoms are less likely to become infected with HIV.

The effectiveness of condoms in prevention of transmission of HIV may be improved by impregnating with chemicals such as nonoxynol-9 which can inactivate the HIV virus. However, there have been reports of some irritation to the vagina from heavy use of nonoxynol-9 treated condoms. When choosing condoms for use by sex workers and other groups you need to evaluate their acceptability.

Guidelines on correct use of a male condom

- When you buy a condom check that the expiry date has not passed and that the outer covering looks in good condition.

- Keep a supply of condoms conveniently at hand either in the home or in your bag. Keep it somewhere cool and where they will not be crushed or exposed to direct sunlight.

- Use a new condom each time you have intercourse.

- Do not test a condom by inflating it or stretching it. Open the packet carefully and be careful of tearing it with sharp fingernails.

- Put the condom on before inserting the penis into the partner. Either the man or the woman can put the condom on the penis.

- Unroll the condom on the erect penis. The condom must be placed with the rolled portion out so that it will unroll properly. The small sack at the end should be pinched to remove the air so that ejaculated semen can collect there.

- If desired, lubricate the outside of the condom using contraceptive jelly or another water-soluble lubricant. Do not use a petroleum-based lubricant such as vaseline as this will weaken the condom.

- After ejaculation, be sure that the condom does not become dislodged from the penis. Hold the rim of the condom firmly against the base of the penis during withdrawal taking care not to spill any semen.

- Dispose of the condom somewhere where children will not find it.

The effectiveness of condoms depend heavily on the man's willingness and ability to use them properly. Men often hold the power in relationships. Women can find it difficult to insist that men use them.

Sex workers may find that their clients refuse to use condoms. There is increasing interest in barrier methods that women can control. One approach that is being explored is the use of 'microbiocides'. These are chemical substances in the form of gels, creams or suppositories that kill HIV and other microorganisms. When placed in the vagina or rectum they should prevent infection with HIV and other sexually transmitted diseases. One of the first to be tried out was nonoxynol-9 which had already been used as an additional protection for condom users. Unfortunately in trials, nonoxyonol-9 has not been shown to reduce infection. Furthermore when used in high concentrations it can irritate the walls of the vagina and may even increase risk of infection. So far, despite extensive testing of other possible chemicals, no effective microbicides have been found.

The female condom is a 17-cm long lubricated polyurethane bag with inner and outer rings. The inner ring can be easily placed in the vagina by the woman and the outer ring rests outside and prevents the condom from slipping entirely inside the vagina. The female condom is manufactured by the Female Health Company under the names

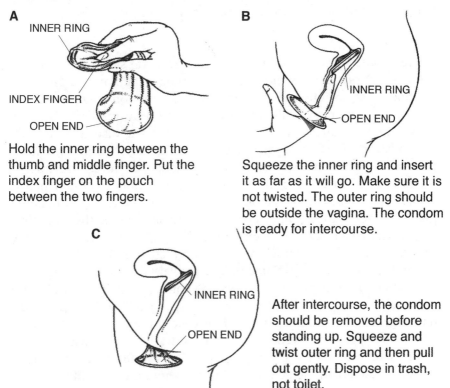

A

INNER RING

INDEX FINGER

OPEN END

Hold the inner ring between the thumb and middle finger. Put the index finger on the pouch between the two fingers.

B

INNER RING

OPEN END

Squeeze the inner ring and insert it as far as it will go. Make sure it is not twisted. The outer ring should be outside the vagina. The condom is ready for intercourse.

C

INNER RING

OPEN END

After intercourse, the condom should be removed before standing up. Squeeze and twist outer ring and then pull out gently. Dispose in trash, not toilet.

Figure 9. The female condom (Courtesy of the Female Health Company)

'Femidon', 'Reality' and 'Femi'. There is evidence both from laboratory and human studies that if used properly it can prevent sexually transmitted diseases. A study in Thailand found that providing both male and female condoms to sex workers in brothels resulted in a greater prevention of sexually transmitted diseases than just providing the male condom.

Responses from the trials in Africa have shown a high level of acceptability for the female condom. Positive points that have emerged include the ability to insert well before intercourse, less slippage and breakage than with the male condom and the ability to use different kinds of lubrication, However negative points that have been found include difficulty that some people find in inserting the condom, discomfort associated with the inner ring, noise during sex and the movement of the condom during sex. Sex workers have responded to the female condom particularly well because they can put it on themselves and do not risk losing male clients by insisting that they wear a condom. Unfortunately the female condom is more expensive than the male condom. Further developments are needed either to lower the price or develop re-usable female condoms.

Safer sex

Some people may be confused by the term safe sex that is used by both AIDS prevention and family planning programmes. However, methods that are effective at preventing conception such as the pill, IUD and diaphragm will not prevent HIV transmission. The safe period in the natural family planning method is also a time when transmission of HIV can take place. Both men and women who have had family planning sterilisation operations can infect others and themselves be infected by HIV. Although it does not contain sperm, semen from men with vasectomies can transmit HIV. The only family planning method that will prevent HIV transmission is the condom.

The term 'safe sex' has been replaced by *safer sex* as few of the low risk activities described above are completely safe although they certainly reduce the risk. Some people are very critical of basing AIDS prevention programmes on safer sex and condom distribution. They see these actions as no substitute for messages such as 'no sex before marriage' or 'one partner for life'. However, there are many people for whom messages of abstinence or faithfulness are unrealistic and for whom safer sex including the use of condoms would be more realistic advice. These might include young people beginning adult life who may not get married for 10 years or more, men and women away from home and sex workers (prostitutes) for whom sex is a vital source of earnings.

The message of abstinence from sex is also not realistic for persons who are infected with HIV and are either symptomless carriers or have symptoms of AIDS. It is not realistic to expect them to abstain from sex. But protection must be provided for their partners.

In practice it is best to combine both approaches. Long-term changes in sexual behaviours are very important and should be the main emphasis for educational programmes. These should be combined with promotion of safer sexual practices that can immediately reduce the risk of transmission of HIV. Guidance should be given to individuals to make the best choice for meeting their own special needs. This is discussed further in the next chapter on counselling.

Prevention of sexually transmitted diseases

As you saw in the previous chapter, the presence of a sexually transmitted disease infection (STD) such as syphilis or chancroid greatly increases the risk of HIV transmission through sexual intercourse. The clearest demonstration of the importance of STDs came from a study in Mwanza, Tanzania that was reported in 1995. That study found that treating STD patients reduced the transmission of HIV by 40% compared with a group that did not receive treatment. Although results of follow-up studies in Rakai, Uganda have not been as clear, the value of treatment of STDs has been clearly demonstrated. In countries where the HIV infection level is still low, STD control is one of the most effective ways of preventing the increase of AIDS.

Unfortunately, despite the widespread prevalence of STDs and their serious nature, the control of STDs often has low importance. The emergence of the AIDS epidemic has led to more effort to control STDs. Many countries have taken the sensible step of combining their AIDS and STD activities into a single reproductive health programme.

Most STDs are easily treated by antibiotics, which have to be chosen carefully to take into account local patterns of antibiotic resistance among the STD-causing microorganisms. Sometimes people delay going for treatment because they do not recognise the symptoms. While the symptoms are easily recognisable in men, they can go unnoticed in women until late in the disease. The early warning signs for action are:

- an itching, soreness or discharge from vagina, penis or anus;
- a sore, lump or rash on genital area or anus;
- an increased frequency in urinating and pain in doing so.

Many countries are responding to the challenge of AIDS by strengthening their STD services and developing public education programmes to promote awareness of symptoms and the importance of early diagnosis and treatment. Special clinics are being opened that provide screening, confidential treatment and counselling on prevention. Counselling should include advice on prevention of AIDS. Condoms should be provided and their use explained. It is becoming routine to screen STD patients for HIV and special counselling should be provided for persons who are found to be HIV antibody positive.

It is important to reach the sexual partners of STD patients – especially the female partners who may not have any symptoms. This is called *partner notification*. As many people find it embarrassing to tell their partners about their STDs, health workers can approach them in confidence – this is called *contact tracing*.

Counselling of STD patients should include the following advice:

● Take all medicines that you have been prescribed to treat the STD. Make sure you complete the full course of treatment. Do not take medicines from other sources.
● Make sure that you do not pass the infection on to anyone else. Do not have sexual intercourse until you are completely cured.
● Come back for a follow-up visit. This way you can be certain that you have been cured.
● If you become reinfected in the future and develop symptoms, go to a trained health worker for treatment.
● Encourage every person that you may have had sexual intercourse with in recent months to go to the clinic for a check up. This is important for the sake of their own health. It also makes sure that they do not pass an infection on to someone else (or even reinfect you). The symptoms of STDs do not always show themselves – especially with women. So even if they feel fine, it's important that they see a health worker.

Even with improved STD services, effort is needed both to ensure that the services are properly used and also to reach infected persons who do not have symptoms. Unfortunately many people delay coming for treatment, take medicines without doctor's advice or go to people who have not yet been trained. The longer a person with a STD delays going to a trained health worker, the more chance there is of developing serious complications.

People may delay going to use STD services for different reasons. They may feel shy about going to a health centre and believe that someone they know will find out about their STD. Women may be reluctant to be examined by a man. People may feel going to government health services is a waste of time because they do not stock the necessary medicines to treat STDs. People then go directly to pharmacists, traditional healers or market traders and buy medicines without consulting a trained health worker. This is dangerous because the drugs prescribed may not be effective and can also lead to antibiotic resistance.

The development of improved STD services has to be accompanied by educational programmes to tell people about these new services and encourage them to come for treatment. Traditional healers have been involved in STD programmes and encouraged to refer patients with STDs to health workers. Training programmes have been given to pharmacists to ensure that inappropriate drugs are not prescribed.

People – especially women – may delay going for treatment simply because they do not have any visible symptoms and are not aware that they are infected. One way of reaching these women is to screen persons who are attending health services for other reasons. It is already normal practice at antenatal clinics to screen pregnant women for STDs – especially syphilis. Health workers at family planning clinics are now also being encouraged to look for signs of STDs while doing gynaecological examinations. These clinic-based methods need to be supplemented by public education to increase awareness of STDs. Any woman who believes that her sexual partner might have an STD should be encouraged to go to a trained health worker for a check up.

The messages of adoption of safer sexual practices including the use of condoms for prevention of AIDS described above will also prevent sexually transmitted diseases. The slow progression from HIV infection to AIDS means that it is difficult to evaluate AIDS education programmes directly by showing a reduction in AIDS cases. A decline in level of sexually transmitted diseases is a very good indicator of the extent to which the public is taking AIDS education seriously. This has been found in studies of various groups such as truck drivers in Tanzania, sex workers in Thailand and homosexual men in USA where increases in condom use has lead to a sharp fall in levels of sexually transmitted diseases.

Prevention of tuberculosis

TB is one of the most common opportunistic infections from AIDS so measures that prevent the transmission of TB will improve the life expectancy of persons with HIV. TB is a contagious disease spread through droplets in air when infected persons cough, sneeze, spit or talk. The BCG immunisation provides protection to infants and very young children but is less effective for adults. Pasteurisation (heat treatment) of milk is carried out in many countries to prevent transmission from cattle to humans. TB is associated with overcrowded and poorly ventilated housing so measures that improve living conditions – especially in urban slums and shanty towns – will have an impact. One group that is increasingly receiving attention is those in prisons, where levels of TB can be up to 100 times greater than in the general population because of overcrowded conditions and lack of treatment facilities.

Tackling poverty and improving living conditions are long-term processes and the main approach to control of TB is to identify and treat all infected cases and thereby reduce the levels of TB bacillus in the environment. WHO estimate that if left untreated, each person with active TB will infect on average between 10 and 15 persons. One of the most important advances in the treatment of TB has been the DOTS strategy involving multi-drug treatment and close supervision to ensure completion of the full course of treatment (see Chapter 3).

Making blood transfusion services safe

Blood transfusion services have received a great deal of attention in national programmes for the prevention and control of AIDS. Testing of blood for HIV is becoming routine and this should greatly reduce the possibility of spread of HIV through donated blood.

Prevention of infection from blood is not easy. Even if testing equipment is available at the blood bank, it can take 3–4 hours to get the results of an ELISA test. In cases of emergencies (such as road traffic accidents) there may not be time to test blood and the risk of possible HIV infection has to be balanced against the certainty of loss of life from the injury. The development of simple and quicker tests could be of great value in these situations.

As explained in the previous chapter it can take 3–12 weeks for a person to develop antibodies to HIV after infection. Blood taken from a person in this early stage will be infectious but will appear negative in tests. This risk is very small but will persist until better tests become available. Hospitals are now reviewing their transfusion practices to give blood only in life-threatening situations.

The potential for reducing the number of blood transfusions was shown in an early study in Zaire. After an intensive campaign, the number of blood transfusions reduced from 16,352 in 1986 to 4531 in 1987. This was achieved without any increase in mortality.

Another way to reduce the risk of transfusing contaminated blood is to discourage potential blood donors who might be HIV positive. Persons whose blood was found to contain antibodies to HIV can be asked not to donate blood again. In countries where heavy use is made of 'professional donors' drawn from poor sections of the community there is increased interest in setting up voluntary blood donor schemes. In some countries leaflets have been distributed to potential donors requesting them not to give blood if they have special characteristics which include: have recently had a sexually transmitted disease or have multiple sex partners. These are called 'donor deferral' programmes. Another approach is to take blood from healthy young persons such as secondary school children where the level of HIV infection is likely to be lower. Whatever approach is taken, it is necessary to provide a counselling service for persons who are found during the testing of blood to be HIV antibody positive or who develop anxieties from the screening questions.

In some countries people may deliberately give blood to find out if they are infected with HIV. This wastes resources because of the demands it makes on blood transfusion services to provide counselling facilities and the cost of drawing infected blood that cannot be used. The best way to solve this problem is to respond to the demand from the community and provide testing facilities. This was the approach adopted in Uganda – as a result between 1989 to 1995 the amount of donated blood at the national blood bank found to contain HIV dropped from 14% to 2% (see next chapter for more details of the Ugandan voluntary counselling and testing programme).

Publicity about AIDS and blood transfusions has led to some people becoming afraid to give blood. Health education messages to the public should stress the safety of giving blood and let the public know what is being done to strengthen the national transfusion services.

Prevention of transmission from mother to child

With studies showing that up to 30% of pregnant women in some countries are infected with HIV, prevention of transmission from mothers to their children becomes an urgent priority. The discovery in 1994 that transmission from mothers to children could be prevented by the drug AZT was a landmark in the struggle against AIDS. In developed countries the number of babies infected with HIV from their mothers has declined to one-tenth and even less as a result of prevention strategies. In developing countries, where the numbers of infected women of childbearing age are much higher, the potential benefits of prevention are considerable. However there are formidable technical, economic and ethical problems involved in prevention of mother-to-child transmission in developing countries.

The spectacular drop in transmission in developed countries has come about through treatment of the pregnant mother and the resulting baby with antiviral drugs and abstinence from breastfeeding. It has been difficult to repeat this successful approach in developing countries. The original drugs used were expensive (about US$1000 per pregnancy) and had to be given repeatedly during pregnancy with monitoring by trained health workers for side effects. Among poor mothers alternatives to breastfeeding, such as bottlefeeding, expose the child to risks of diarrhoea, dehydration, malnutrition and infections. The risk of mother-to-child transmission can also be reduced by delivery through Cesarean section. However the lack of facilities for safe surgical procedures and the costs/risks involved make this an inappropriate option for most situations.

A way forward involving the three components described below is beginning to emerge by which prevention of transmission from mother to child can be implemented in developing countries.

Treatment of the infected mother

In developed countries a pregnant woman might be offered AZT from 14 weeks of pregnancy and the baby given the drug for the first 6 weeks. This is expensive and requires careful monitoring of the health of the mother and child. Intensive research is underway to find simpler procedures. Promising alternatives being tested involve giving AZT later in pregnancy, in smaller (and therefore cheaper) doses and in combination with other drugs. A recent development in 1999 was the demonstration in a trial in Uganda that substantial impact on transmission could be achieved by a single dose of the drug nevirapine to the pregnant mother at onset of labour and also to the newborn baby. This treatment costs about US$4. It is likely that substantial advances will be made in the next few years in the cost and feasibility of treatment procedures for prevention of mother-to-child transmission.

Reduction in risks from prolonged breastfeeding

The risks of HIV transmission through breastfeeding have to be set against the benefits of breastfeeding. A recent review by WHO concluded that in developing countries a baby who was not breast-fed was six times more likely to die from infectious diseases. This risk would be even greater for poorer homes who do not have the facilities for hygienic food preparation. In 1997 UNAIDS, in partnership with WHO and UNICEF, issued a joint policy statement recommending that mothers infected with HIV should abstain from breastfeeding and use alternatives such as formula feed or modified milk from cows, goats or other animals. If this is not realistic, mothers may choose from the following three strategies:

1. Exclusive breastfeeding of the baby for the first few months only, to ensure that the baby gets the maximum protective benefit. Then stop breastfeeding and start to feed with either formula feed or, for the older infant aged 4–6 months, with weaning food that is rich in nutrients and energy.
2. The mother expressing her milk which is then heat treated and fed to the baby. (Pasteurization at 62.5°C for 30 minutes will inactivate most of the HIV.)
3. Wet nursing of the baby by a woman who has been tested HIV negative.

UNAIDS has issued guidelines for health workers and policy makers that provide detailed descriptions of different possible feeding strategies. The first of the above three is probably the most realistic for many situations – but even that is not easy to implement. Exclusive means *only* breast milk and *no other foods or drinks*. There is some evidence that additional foods might cause irritation of the child's digestive tract and therefore increase likelihood of HIV transmission. Mothers will need continued support to prevent breastfeeding problems such as cracked nipples. At the point of transition to solid food, advice should be given on appropriate feeding and the need for: i) hygiene such as hand washing before food preparation, and after handling children's faeces; ii) the importance of cooking food thoroughly, covering and serving fresh and not leaving it to stand; iii) the preparation and use of oral rehydration solution when the child gets diarrhoea.

Other possible actions for reduction of mother-to-child transmission

There are two further actions that could reduce the transmission from mother-to-child – cleansing of the birth canal and changes in sexual behaviour.

As described in the previous chapter some transmission of HIV takes place during passage of the baby through the birth canal. Preliminary results from clinical trials in Malawi found that cleansing the birth canal with the antiseptic chlorhexidine reduced HIV transmission when the membranes had been ruptured for a long time, but had no impact for normal deliveries. However, despite its lack of impact on HIV transmission, the procedure of cleansing of the birth canal would seem worth adopting because the study found it had a major impact reducing other infections during childbirth. It is hoped that there will be more developments on this procedure in future.

If the woman is exposed to further infection during pregnancy, the risk of transmission to the child is increased. It is likely that transmission from the mother to the child can be further reduced if women abstain from sex or use a condom during pregnancy.

Voluntary counselling and testing for women

As can be seen from the discussion above, the steps needed to reduce mother-to-child transmission are not straightforward. In order to implement the above measures a woman must know her HIV status and then be provided the necessary information and support to make the best decision for herself and her child. Advice needs to take into account the needs of the mother as well as risks to the child. For example some mothers will be reluctant to adopt alternatives to breastfeeding because of a genuine fear that it will serve as a visible signal to family and community that they are HIV positive. They might then face discrimination and victimisation. Another problem that has been found is that women may find it difficult to say no when asked to take an HIV test. They then take the test but not return to find out the results.

Prevention of mother-to-child transmission will therefore not only require an adequate health care infrastructure for antenatal care, delivery and essential medicines but also an expansion of facilities for voluntary counselling and testing for women and an active programme of public education to encourage women to use these facilities. This would need to be accompanied by legal, economic and social measures that protect HIV-infected women against discrimination. The importance of human rights is discussed later in this chapter and counselling of women is considered in Chapter 6.

Injections and skin piercing procedures

The AIDS epidemic has led all countries to review their immunisation procedures to reduce the possibility of spread of HIV through contaminated needles and syringes.

In some countries this has involved increasing the supply of disposable syringes. This reduces the risk of transmission of HIV to other patients and also the risk of needlestick injuries to health workers by eliminating the need to take syringes apart for sterilisation. Whenever an injection is given some blood will be drawn from the needle into the chamber so it is not enough just to change the needle, the whole syringe should be changed. Other countries are encouraging the use of low-cost plastic syringes that can be steam sterilised. Simple sterilising units have been developed and are being promoted by UNICEF and WHO. In situations of acute shortages, the temptation to reuse disposable syringes can be strong. Practices to prevent re-use such as bending over the needlepoint are even more dangerous because they increase the risk of needlestick injury. Attempts are being made to develop 'self-destruct' syringes which can only be used once. It is also important to make sure that syringes are properly disposed of, e.g. by burying deep in the ground where they cannot be found and re-used.

The difficulty in ensuring sterilisation or adequate disposable of syringes has led to efforts to replace, whenever possible, injections with oral doses. However, many communities attach higher value to injections and public education is needed to make oral medicines more acceptable.

Traditional birth attendants may sometimes use unsterilised blades to cut the umbilical cord, which can lead to neonatal tetanus and infection with HIV. There have been many programmes to train traditional birth attendants in improved maternity care and the risk of HIV infection makes this even more important.

Many programmes are beginning to work with traditional healers to ensure that activities such as circumcision, facial scarification and other skin-piercing activities are carried out using sterile blades.

Injections by injecting drug users

In countries where there is a problem of persons injecting drugs, extensive programmes have been mounted to prevent the spread of HIV. The key messages are 'Don't use drugs' and 'Don't inject drugs'.

It is very difficult to eliminate the problem of drug abuse through law enforcement and the police alone. A realistic approach is to recognise that drug injection will be difficult to control and promote the concept of *harm reduction*. This involves intensive education among drug injectors to discourage the sharing of needles and promote the practice of sterilising their needles – or 'works' – in bleach solution. Some countries have introduced programmes where drug injectors are provided free sterile syringes that they can use and then exchange for new ones. Needle exchange programmes have been successfully introduced in Europe and the United States through out-reach programmes in the community as well as in institutional settings such as prisons. Another harm-reduction approach being explored is to encourage drug injectors to change from injectable drugs such as heroin to others such as methadone which can be taken by mouth. The lesson drawn from these programmes is that harm-reduction strategies should be accompanied by counselling on safer sex, provision of condoms and the development of a supportive environment by police and other law enforcement agencies.

It is also important to complement this harm-reduction strategy with practical programmes to provide treatment/counselling to help injecting drug users to overcome their addiction, as well as drug education programmes in schools and among the general public. The need for public education on drugs is particularly important in countries where drug injection is only just beginning to emerge as a problem and there is low awareness of the dangers of drugs.

Promoting safe practices by health workers

A list of basic guidelines for health workers to prevent infection at work is given below. All workers in health care settings, including cleaners, sweepers and nurse orderlies, should be briefed on these precautions. The main emphasis should be on avoidance of contact with blood and body fluids such as pus and semen. Most of these are the standard precautions that should be applied, not just against HIV, but to protect against a range of infectious diseases such as hepatitis.

These precautions should be applied to blood and body fluids from all patients, not only from those who are known to have HIV infection or AIDS. Other patients may be carriers of HIV without it being realised and their blood and fluids could be infectious.

Health workers often have to work under difficult conditions where supplies of protective equipment, such as gloves, are limited. These issues of resources and funding are receiving serious attention in the national plans that have been established in most countries.

Fortunately, as was discussed in the previous chapter, there have been very few cases where health workers have been infected with HIV during their work. There is no risk from casual (i.e. non-sexual) contact with AIDS patients, and these patients do not have to be isolated. It is important to treat AIDS patients and carriers of HIV as normally as possible in the hospital and dispel the myths and fears that people have about the disease. The care of AIDS patients will be discussed further in the next chapter.

Recently there has been discussion on *post-exposure prevention* – the giving of drugs such as AZT to health workers who have accidentally been exposed to HIV. In some hospitals in Europe and North America this has become routine practice. However the evidence to support its effectiveness is limited, and as discussed in Chapter 3, administration of anti-HIV drugs have to be carefully monitored for side effects. While post-exposure prevention might become more widely available in the future, primary prevention through the avoidance of exposure to HIV remains the most realistic and appropriate option at present for most situations.

As discussed in Chapter 4 health workers who are HIV antibody positive are of little risk to patients and can continue to work. However, HIV positive health workers who are in contact with tuberculosis patients have an increased risk of developing TB. They are one of the groups for which it would be highly appropriate to offer anti-tuberculosis drugs as preventive therapy (see Chapter 3).

Precautions by health workers to prevent HIV transmission

Protect existing wounds and prevent new wounds:
Cover exposed cuts and abrasions, especially on the hands and fingers, with waterproof dressings.
Take care to prevent puncture wounds, cuts and abrasions from used needles and glassware. If an accident occurs, treat immediately by encouraging bleeding and washing with soap and water.

Prevent direct contact with infected material:
Wear the normal protective clothing such as uniforms and overalls.
As well as the normal protective clothing, wear gloves and apron when there is a possibility of direct contact with blood, other body fluids or contaminated articles.
Avoid blood or contaminated articles coming in contact with parts of your body with cuts, sores or chapped skin.

Dispose of spillages and contaminated materials safely
Wash your hands and any other exposed parts of your body immediately after contact with contaminated material.

Dispose of wastes including needles and broken glass safely
Make sure that all clinical material, e.g. dressings, soiled clothing, placenta etc. are disinfected and disposed of. Incineration is the best method for disposal but if this is not possible then the materials should be buried in deep pits and covered with disinfectant or lime. All contaminated reusable linen should be decontaminated by autoclaving or boiling before washing by the laundry.
Put needles, broken glass and other sharp objects in special containers (plastic

---

bottles can be adapted for this) and do not put them in plastic bags where they can cause injury and infection. HIV is fragile and destroyed at 56°C so boiling for 20 minutes, autoclaving, steam or pressure cooking will destroy the virus.

Control surface contamination

Any surfaces contaminated by spillages of blood and body fluids should be washed and disinfected. Many disinfectants such as chlorine (5 g per litre) or household bleach (one part per 10 parts water) will kill HIV, but ethanol and industrial methylated spirits are not suitable for cleaning surfaces because of their high evaporation rate.

Public health measures

Testing and screening for HIV

Testing specific groups or the general public for HIV can provide valuable information on the levels of HIV infection. If testing is repeated after some time, we can learn about the rate of spread of HIV. Blood for transfusion services should be tested for HIV to protect the recipients. People who are worried that they may be at risk from AIDS may ask to have an antibody test. These are all reasonable actions provided that confidentiality about test results is maintained and counselling is provided for the persons who are found to be HIV antibody positive.

Another policy adopted by some countries is to demand HIV antibody tests from persons wishing to travel to their country as visitors, immigrants or students. This is not an effective method of control – a person may be antibody negative on a test but be in the window period and still be carrying the virus. In 1992 the World Health Assembly passed a resolution agreeing that there is no public health rationale for measures, such as mandatory screening, that arbitrarily limit individual rights. UNAIDS strongly supports the view that a person's HIV positive status should not be a barrier to his or her right to travel.

Some people have suggested that screening programmes should be carried out to identify all persons with HIV. The implications of this should be carefully considered. If a person is found to have HIV what action should follow? If counselling and treatment were provided then this might seem sensible. However, there are those who would like to isolate HIV antibody positive persons in remand homes, gaols or special colonies. This would reinforce the stigma and prejudice against AIDS patients and HIV carriers and in the long term make prevention and control of the disease much more difficult.

In a climate of fear and prejudice about HIV and AIDS many people may feel that it is not in their best interest to be tested and found HIV positive. However, HIV testing is important for protecting blood supplies and monitoring (surveillance) of the level of HIV infection in the community. For surveillance and screening the most realistic approach is *unlinked anonymous testing* in which the person's identity is removed from the test sample so it is not possible to identify persons with a positive test result.

Even 5 years ago the benefits of being tested for HIV were not very obvious. However, the availability of combination therapy and measures to prevent the mother-to-child transmission has changed this situation. There are now real advantages to knowing if one is infected with HIV both for one's own health and for prevention of transmission to one's partner and baby. The development of voluntary counselling and testing services and the promotion of their uptake by the community is now seen as an important approach for prevention. More information is provided in the next chapter on counselling.

Ethical issues, human rights and the stigma of AIDS

Dealing with AIDS involves confronting many difficult decisions including the following:

- Should we test a person's blood without his or her knowledge or permission?
- Should a person be compelled to have an HIV test?
- Should people be denied entry to a country if they are HIV antibody positive?
- Should every person coming for surgery or deliveries be made to have an HIV test?
- Should a health worker be forced against his/her will to care for an AIDS patient?
- Should a doctor be forced to report centrally if he finds out that a patient is HIV antibody positive?
- If an HIV antibody positive person refuses to behave responsibly in his/her sexual relations, should force be used to restrain him/her?
- Should condoms be made available to children without consent of parents?
- Should vaccines or drugs be tested on sections of the community if their safety and effectivness is not proven?
- Is it right to enrol people in trials for drugs or vaccines if it means that they may only receive a placebo (control pill with no drug) and be denied a possible life-saving measure?

- Should access to combination therapy for AIDS be made available to some people and not others? How would the decision on who receives treatment be made?
- Should access to treatment depend on the person's ability to pay for the drugs?

For many of these issues there are no answers that are universally appropriate. Each society has to make a decision that is socially, economically, politically and culturally acceptable. Many of these involve ethical decisions on the rights of individuals compared with that of society as a whole. The fears and anxieties aroused by AIDS can lead to people calling for extreme repressive measures that restrict human freedom without contributing very much to preventing the problem. Debates about public control measures are often influenced by prejudice against minority groups such as homosexuals, sex workers or injecting drug users.

In recognition of the importance of human rights and AIDS the World Health Assembly of the United Nations in 1988 passed a resolution calling on all its member states to:

Foster a spirit of understanding and compassion for HIV-infected people and people with AIDS through information, education and social support programmes;

Protect the human rights and dignity of HIV-infected people and people with AIDS, and of members of population groups, and to avoid discriminatory action and stigmatization of them in the provision of services, employment and travel;

Ensure the confidentiality of HIV testing and to promote the availability of confidential counselling and other support services to HIV-infected people and people with AIDS.

This declaration led to a series of international meetings exploring the human rights implications of HIV and AIDS. A comprehensive set of 12 guidelines were developed in 1996 at the Second International Consultation on HIV/AIDS and Human Rights jointly hosted by UNAIDS and the Office of the UN High Commissioner for Human Rights. The guidelines included recommendations for reforming laws and legal support services focusing on anti-discrimination, protection of public health and the improvement of the status of women, children and marginalised groups. In implementing these changes the declaration recognised the need for improving the capacity of governments to take on responsibility for dealing with the issues and also called for increased non-governmental organisation (NGO), private sector and community involvement in the preservation of human rights.

In looking at AIDS we can draw lessons from the shameful history of leprosy where people were stigmatised for an affliction and isolated in leper colonies. We now know that leprosy is not very infectious but the stigma of leprosy remains as a barrier to prompt action. Lack of compassion and tolerance towards HIV carriers and AIDS cases will only drive the disease underground and make it much more difficult to control. We now have guidelines – the challenge is to put them into practice!

AIDS and the law

The need to tackle the AIDS epidemic has led to many countries re-examining their legal system and changing laws to protect human rights, tackle stigma and support prevention and control activities. In some countries NGOs, such as the AIDS Law Project at Wits University, South Africa, have been established to campaign on human rights and provide legal help to people in the community affected by AIDS.

Laws that need abolishing are those which discriminate against people and make it difficult to develop effective control policies. These include: laws which make homosexuality, prostitution or drug injection a criminal offence and interfere with educational interventions; censorship and broadcasting laws which make it difficult to carry out public education on safe sex; laws that allow HIV testing without consent, detention or restriction of immigration of people with HIV.

Laws that need to be introduced to support AIDS control measures include: laws that give rights to privacy, confidentiality and prevent discrimination in employment, access to health care and housing against people with HIV or their family and friends; laws that protect the rights of persons with HIV in the workplace.

The increase in the numbers of children orphaned by AIDS has pointed to the need for improved laws to protect the human rights of children affected by AIDS – especially their right to inheritance, schooling, health care, freedom from violence and exploitation. The basic rights of children are set out in the Convention of the Rights of the Child which was adopted by the United Nations in 1989 and has now been ratified by most countries of the world (except United States and Somalia). Some countries have taken the safeguards for children further by introducing specific policies concerning AIDS orphans. In Zimbabwe an orphans policy was approved by their Cabinet in 1999 containing the four main tenets below:

- Care of orphans in institutions should be only a last resort and should be temporary. Emphasis should be on community-based care.

- All children, including orphans, should receive education, and there should be laws and guidelines to enforce this right.
- The property rights of orphans should be safeguarded by legislation.
- The care and protection of orphans must comply with the Convention on the Rights of the Child and the African Charter on the Rights and Welfare of the Child.

National action for control of AIDS

The key body for directing national effort in the control and prevention of AIDS is the National AIDS Control Programme. This will have involvement of government ministries including health, education, social welfare, information, women's affairs, youth and sports and defence. In addition a range of NGOs may be involved including bodies such as Red Cross and Red Crescent societies, family planning associations and other agencies. Many countries have set up short-term and later medium-term 3–5 year plans with the typical components shown below.

Typical components for national actions

- **Surveillance and research:** setting up a targeted surveillance to monitor the development of the HIV/AIDS epidemic and provide information for planning, monitoring and evaluating prevention programmes.
- **Education, communication and social mobilisation:** educational programmes directed at general public and specific target groups in a range of settings including community, workplace and schools.
- **Condom promotion:** improving quality of condoms and promoting the use of condoms.
- **Blood safety:** strengthening national blood transfusion system through upgrading, improved HIV testing facilities, training and expansion of voluntary blood donation system.
- **Strengthening of health and social provision by government and NGOs:** counselling for HIV infected individuals and AIDS cases; care and support for AIDS orphans; establishment of policies/services for testing, treatment and setting up of home care services. Strengthening of STD services. Review of national essential drug lists to take into account treatment needs for STDs and HIV/AIDS. Training of field staff.
- **Actions to safeguard human rights and remove the stigma attached to AIDS:** Review of national legislation to counter discrimination, guidelines for police and courts, guidelines on confidentiality.

The experiences of most countries have pointed to the importance of broadening the base of AIDS prevention activities to include other reproductive health activities, especially the treatment and control of sexually transmitted diseases and the delivery of family planning. In addition these programmes have emphasised the need to widen the range of organisations involved in AIDS control beyond health to involve other sectors including education, social welfare, industry and agriculture as well as the involvement of NGOs, which include missions, charities and voluntary organisations. A third lesson has been the importance of gaining political commitment from policy makers to support AIDS control activities and introduce supportive legislation to protect human rights and remove discrimination

Prevention and political will

The advances that have been made in recent years have shown that prevention programmes can make a difference. A vital ingredient for success is political commitment at the community, national and international level. Unfortunately in many countries there is still a big gap between the rhetoric of speeches and policy documents and the reality of action where programmes are poorly funded and jealousy over departmental boundary areas take priority over true collaboration. It would be wrong, however, to put all the blame on national governments. Programmes of structural adjustment and the burden of debt repayments have placed severe restrictions on the resources that governments can allocate to AIDS.

In his appropriately titled speech 'Time to Turn the Tide' delivered at the XII International AIDS Conference at Durban, South Africa, Dr Peter Piot, Director of UNAIDS stated "We have come to Durban to break the silence – to break the silence, stigma indifference and ignorance surrounding the AIDS epidemic…". He called for the amount spent on fighting AIDS to be increased ten times to at least 3 billion dollars a year. The international community has a responsibility to increase its support to meet this challenge. While it seems a large sum, in reality it a small amount and easily affordable. It is less than the budget of a medium size company in Europe and equivalent to just 4 cents of every US$100 earned in the developed countries. It is only a fifth of the 15 billion dollars that African countries are paying per year in debt repayments (a good start would be for the developed countries to cancel more of these debts!). Expressed in another way, if divided equally in the world the amount being asked for is only 50 cents per person in the world – the cost of a can of fizzy drink – a small price to pay for tackling one of the greatest scourges of modern times!

6. Counselling and support for persons with AIDS and HIV

This chapter will explore the kinds of services needed to help persons who are worried that they have AIDS, are to have an HIV antibody test, have been diagnosed as having HIV or have symptoms of AIDS.

Counselling is an essential component of services for persons with HIV and AIDS. It is also an important approach to use with any person who is worried about AIDS and wants advice on the best way of reorienting his or her lifestyle to reduce the risk of becoming infected with HIV. A range of services including sexually transmitted diseases clinics, programmes with sex workers, family planning clinics, hospitals, schools, colleges, social welfare, occupational health all need to consider developing some sort of counselling provision.

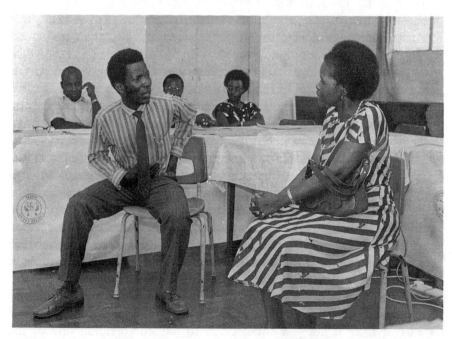

Figure 10. Training health workers in counselling on AIDS in Uganda using role play

The counselling process

In traditional advice giving, the health worker is often trying to persuade a person to follow a particular course of action. Counselling is a process that goes beyond simply giving information but involves helping people to make decisions and giving them the confidence to put their decisions into practice.

Counselling is based on the following assumptions:

- Counselling should consider the psychosocial, financial and spiritual needs of the client.
- Everything said during a counselling session should be treated as strictly confidential.
- Any information provided should be based on the best available understanding of the subject, accurate and clearly put.
- The emphasis should be that of promoting informed decision making by the client.
- The client has the right to choose his or her own actions.

One useful way of remembering the basic principles of counselling is the word **GATHER** (adapted from Population Reports).

G Greet the person. Put them at ease, show respect and trust. Emphasise the confidential nature of the discussion.

A Ask about their problem and LISTEN to what they say. Encourage them to bring out their anxieties, worries and needs. Assess their present degree of risk behaviour. Determine their access to support and help in their family and community. Find out what steps they have already taken to deal with the situation. Encourage them to express their feelings in their own words. Show respect and tolerance to what they say and do not pass judgement. Actively listen and show that you are interested and paying attention. Encourage them through helpful questions.

T Tell them any relevant information they need. Provide accurate and specific information in reply to their questions. Give information on how they can reduce their risk of becoming infected with HIV. Demonstrate the use of condoms. Explain the HIV test and what it detects. Keep your language simple, repeat important points and ask questions to check that the important points are understood. Provide the important information in a leaflet that they can take away.

H Help them make decisions. Explore the various alternatives. Raise issues they may not have thought of. Be careful of letting your own views, values and prejudices influence the advice you give. Ensure that it is their own decision and not one that you have imposed. Help them make a plan of action.

E Explain any misunderstandings. Ask questions to check understanding of important points. Ask the person to repeat back in his/her own words the key points you have made.

R Return to follow up. Arrange for a follow-up visit or referral to other agencies. If a follow-up visit is not necessary, give the name of someone who they can contact it they have need for help.

You can use these guidelines to assess the effectiveness of your advice giving and counselling activities. In addition you should consider the various issues raised in Chapter 7 concerning understanding the community and selection of messages. A difficulty all of us have is to avoid imposing our own views on others. We need to try to understand our own values, opinions and prejudices so that we feel comfortable about talking about sex and do not impose our own values on others.

The 'worried well'

With the expansion of public education programmes on AIDS, many people develop fears and anxieties about contracting HIV or AIDS. This fear may have a real basis, e.g. a visit to a sex worker, a 'one-night stand' or from some imagined risk. Many symptoms of AIDS are non-specific such as weight loss, diarrhoea and swollen lymph nodes and it is easy to imagine that one has AIDS.

Anyone with anxieties about AIDS should be taken seriously. You should discuss with them the reasons for their fears and assess the degree of risk that they may have contracted HIV. If the risk is unlikely, you can reassure them. If there has been a real risk, you can discuss the desirability of them having the HIV test (but see below about pre-test counselling). In either case you need to explain how they can reduce the risk of becoming infected with HIV through adopting the safer sexual practices described in Chapter 5.

Many countries have set up telephone counselling services or 'AIDS hotlines'. These are often run by trained volunteers and offer confidential advice to anyone who calls.

Pre-test counselling

Besides the 'worried well' there are other groups to whom it might be appropriate to offer an HIV test. These include:

- persons who feel that they are at risk through their behaviour,
- persons who have been diagnosed with sexually transmitted diseases,
- injecting drug users,
- tuberculosis patients,
- people who have received unscreened blood,
- couples wishing to get married,
- travellers requiring the HIV antibody test for a visa,
- victims of rape attacks.

You should read this section along with the discussion on the biology of the HIV antibody test in Chapter 2 and the role of screening as a preventive health measure in Chapter 5. The purpose of pre-test counselling is to ensure that the decision to have the HIV test is one of *informed consent*. This involves explaining to the person exactly what the test reveals as well as some of the shortcomings. Whether or not a person should be advised to have a test depends heavily on the particular situation. If a person has a test and it proves positive what impact would it have? In many countries a person who has had a positive result on an HIV test will face many problems. These include discrimination, social isolation, desertion by their spouse and losing their job. It is important to reassure the person that the test result will be confidential and not revealed to employers or others.

Some counsellors consider that it is important to give pre-test counselling to parents of babies who are suspected of having AIDS. This makes it easier to break the news to the parents if the baby is found to have AIDS and the mother and probably the father are infected.

If the person is the victim of a rape attack her counselling needs will go beyond that of the implications of HIV. Counselling will need to provide emotional, medical and legal support. Many countries have women's rape crisis centres who are well placed to provide specific help.

If a person definitely wants to have the HIV test they should be allowed to do so. However, the outcome of pre-test counselling may be that they decide not to have the test and this decision should also be respected. Whether or not a person decides to go ahead with the test, they should be counselled on personal behaviour to reduce the risk of contracting HIV and passing it on to others.

Post-test counselling

A negative result

The relief of discovering that the test is negative can be a powerful motivating force to adopt safer sexual practices. Even if the results are negative, you should give advice on low risk behaviours to avoid future infection. It should also be explained that a person can still be infected but have not yet developed antibodies. A second test 3 months later is necessary to establish that the person is free of infection.

A positive result

If the test is positive you will certainly need to counsel the person. Do not raise unnecessary anxiety about a positive ELISA test before it is confirmed by another test such as the Western blot. A person who has had pre-test counselling will have had some preparation in the earlier counselling session. However, if the person has not received pre-test counselling he or she may be completely unprepared. This can be the case when the positive result has arisen following routine testing of donated blood by the blood transfusion service or screening of cases at antenatal and sexually transmitted disease clinics.

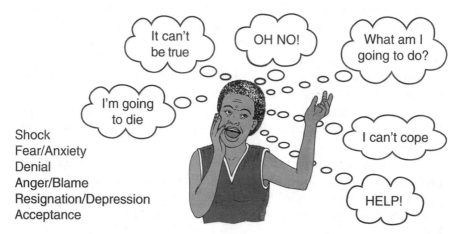

Figure 11. Common reaction stages to being diagnosed as infected with HIV or AIDS

If a positive result is confirmed you will have to break the news. Some of the feelings that a person may have on discovering that they are infected or have AIDS are shown in Figure 11. At first the person may be so shocked at the news that he or she may not absorb necessary information you will need to give. You will need to reassure them that they do not have AIDS and might expect many years of normal life before the possible onset of AIDS. In particular you will have to get over the following:

- Being infected with HIV is not the same as having the disease AIDS.
- HIV is not spread by normal social contact so most normal routines in the family, community and at work can be continued.
- There can be a period of up to 10 years between infection and onset of AIDS and it is not possible to predict exactly how long this period will last in an individual person.
- It is important to maintain your general health. You should see a heath worker if you have any symptoms of ill health including possible AIDS-related opportunistic infections.
- You must take precautions in your sexual contact with others to reduce the risk of spread of HIV. This means adopting safer sexual practices including use of the condom (see prevention guidelines in Chapter 5).
- Adopting safer sex practices will also benefit your own health. Repeated attacks of other STDs and re-infections with other strains of HIV may accelerate the progress of the disease in an individual.
- You should take actions to reduce the risk of passing HIV to others including not donating blood, semen or organs and care in dealing with any spillages of blood.

The first counselling session usually concentrates on breaking the news and providing specific information. A follow-up session is arranged a few weeks later where questions are answered and the key information above is repeated. You will need to provide comfort and support to help deal with feelings of guilt and anxiety.

In addition you will need to help the HIV antibody positive person to make some important decisions. One important decision is who they should tell about their HIV status. There are very few people who need to know. Hasty decisions should be avoided because of the prejudice and discrimination that surrounds AIDS in most societies. You will also have to discuss the need to inform their sexual partner. This will not be an easy task and in some situations will involve confessions of unfaithfulness or bisexuality. You will need to arrange meetings with sexual partners to provide counselling about the advisability of having the HIV test.

The next group of decisions to be made will be regarding changes in lifestyle and sexual behaviour: to reduce the risk of receiving further infections of HIV; and of passing HIV on to others. You will need to help the person choose which low-risk behaviours are realistic and appropriate to their personal situation.

One difficult issue is whether an unmarried HIV antibody positive person should get married in future. Social pressures to get married can be very strong. However, if they do decide to get married, you will have to advise on safer sex practices to ensure that their spouse does not become infected. They also should clearly understand the risks of infecting their future children with HIV (see also the discussion below on counselling of women).

Another set of decisions will centre around present and future needs for health care. If the person has tuberculosis (TB) it would be appropriate to initiate treatment based on the DOTS approach. If he or she does not show symptoms of TB it may be appropriate to begin preventive therapy – especially for those who have a positive skin test for TB or who are in regular contact with persons with TB such as health workers or relatives of TB patients (see discussion of TB in Chapter 3). The person should also be advised of the importance of seeking early health care on health problems in general or specific conditions such as sexually transmitted infections, opportunistic infections or pregnancy.

Further counselling sessions can provide a valuable opportunity to address both broader psychosocial issues as well as to identify and act upon any health care needs that might develop. It is helpful to arrange meetings with other HIV antibody positive persons. These meetings provide valuable opportunities to share feelings and concerns and to overcome the sense of isolation. In Britain, infected persons have set up a self-help group called 'Body Positive' to provide mutual support and promote the rights of HIV antibody positive persons. Other examples of self-help groups are 'Positive People' in Goa, India and 'TASO' in Uganda.

Voluntary counselling and testing (VCT) programme

In many countries there is a movement to support the setting up of voluntary counselling and testing programmes. In the early days of the AIDS epidemic it was still not clear whether it was beneficial for a person to know his or her HIV status. However, the emergence of combination therapy for both the treatment of persons with HIV and the prevention of mother-child transmission now provide clear benefits to knowing one's HIV status.

In Uganda the setting up of voluntary counselling and testing programme services was in response to the demand from some members of the community to know if they were infected with HIV. People were deliberately giving blood just to find out their HIV status. This was felt to be inappropriate use of blood transfusion services, which had to discard large amounts of contaminated blood and did not have the trained staff to provide the counselling required for those who were found to be HIV positive.

Over an 8-year period from 1990 Uganda's VCT programme grew from one AIDS Information Centre in Kampala in 1990 to a network of 35 VCT sites in hospitals and health centres throughout the country – providing counselling to more than 40,000 persons a year. About half the clients were young people between the ages of 20 and 29 – many of whom came because they were deciding whether to get married or start a relationship. More recently, the onset of pregnancy has been a reason for women to come to be tested.

Initially the counselling process required two visits separated by 2 weeks – the time for the test results to become available. This had the disadvantage that clients might not return for the follow-up. In some of their centres, rapid HIV tests were introduced so that results could be given back on the same day. This one-day VCT involves five stages: anonymous registration, orientation and test decision counselling (5–15 minutes in both group and individual sessions), drawing of blood, prevention counselling (45 minute group session while the test is carried out) and giving of the test results and counselling (5–15 minutes individual session). Both the clients who are found to be HIV anti-body positive and also those who are negative are encouraged to join the post-test club run by the VCT centre which provides support activities. During the counselling clients are provided information on family planning and sexually transmitted diseases and provided with condoms. In addition to HIV, blood is also tested for syphilis and any clients found positive for syphilis are provided with treatment.

The counsellors come from backgrounds in health, teaching and social work. Their training takes place over a 6-month period which includes both counselling skills, workshops and supervised work experience. The counsellors are supported by volunteers who are members of post-test clubs who have undergone a short training course.

The high and continuing demand for VCT in Uganda indicates that the services are meeting a need. Further evidence for the benefits of VCT come from follow-up evaluations of clients, which show that both HIV positive and negative clients increased condom use after VCT. The post-test clubs are the basis for educational activities among the members and surrounding community through drama activities, peer education and social marketing of condoms.

There are two main issues that need to be considered when adapting the Uganda VCT model to other situations. Of particular importance is the cost of the service which in 1997 was US$13.39 per client. Initially the service was provided free but to cope with the expanded demand charges have been introduced. To minimise the negative impact of charges the VCT service is free on certain days, e.g. World AIDS Day, International Women's Day and even Valentines Day! Special provisions are also made for those who clearly cannot afford the charges.

Another problem comes from the shift to one day sessions. Unfortunately, as discussed in Chapter 2, most of the rapid tests require refrigeration and are expensive when only a few tests are carried out at a time. Hopefully this problem will disappear with improvements in testing methods.

In the early stages of the AIDS epidemic there was no real advantage of public education programmes to motivate people to come for testing. Now that we have combination therapies and the knowledge of how to reduce the risk of mother-to-child transmission there are definite advantages to both the individual and society of knowing one's HIV status. Putting this knowledge into practice will require a large expansion of VCT facilities.

Counselling women of childbearing age

A woman of childbearing age has special needs. The aim of counselling is to help her take the necessary actions to ensure that she does not become infected with HIV. If she does become infected, the aim of counselling is to protect her own health, that of her sexual partner and family including any future children. You would need to raise the following topics.

- Disclosure of results to male partners and/or to other significant family or community members: advantages and risks
- The effect of pregnancy on HIV infection.
- The risk of transmission to the baby during pregnancy, delivery and breastfeeding
- Termination of pregnancy options

- Treatment options during pregnancy
- Interventions available to attempt to prevent mother-to-child transmission
- Infant feeding options: the advantages and disadvantages of breastfeeding; safe alternatives to breastfeeding
- The need for follow-up of both mother and child
- Whether to have further pregnancies and contraceptive options

It can be particularly difficult for a woman to tell her partner that she is infected with HIV. He may blame her when it is as likely that he may have become infected first and passed it on to her. So some counsellors, with the permission of the woman, try to arrange it so that both partners are informed at the same time. This way it will be the counsellor, not the woman, who breaks the news to the other partner.

One of the most difficult issues is whether an HIV positive woman should have further children who may become infected with HIV. The transmission of HIV from a mother to her baby was discussed in Chapter 4. Chapter 5 discussed the difficult issues opened up with recent developments in understanding of the contribution of breastfeeding and in the use of combination therapy to prevent mother-to-child transmission.

Some people feel that an HIV positive woman should be given advice on family planning and have no further pregnancies. Others feel that this is unrealistic in societies where childbearing is important for the status of a woman. If an HIV infected woman does go on to become pregnant it is important that counselling is provided to help her make an informed choice about taking antiviral drugs (if available) and about safe alternatives to breastfeeding. As discussed in Chapter 5 these are not easy choices and will depend both on her circumstances and the availability of suitable health care and support. It is increasingly realised that counselling about HIV and the opportunity to be tested should be provided to all pregnant women as part of regular antenatal care.

Sometimes it is only discovered that a woman is HIV antibody positive when her child has been brought in sick and has been diagnosed as suffering from AIDS. Telling a mother that her child has AIDS is a particularly difficult and sensitive task. You have to tell her that her child has a fatal illness. You also have to tell her further bad news: that she is also infected even though she may be feeling well at that time; that she will always be infectious; that there is a high risk that she will infect her future babies; and that her husband may also be infected. She will not be able to understand all this at once. She will need several counselling sessions.

Because of these problems, it is important to provide pre-test counselling to parents before testing a child for HIV so they are prepared for the possibility of a positive result.

In a recent review of 11 studies, UNAIDS found the average rates of HIV infection to be five times higher in teenage girls than boys. Counselling infected adolescents poses special challenges. It will be important to ensure that the adolescent is not discriminated against and can continue school. Confidentiality should be protected and counselling would need to address the issue of whether to inform the child's parents.

The AIDS patient

Often, the confirmation of HIV-antibody positive status takes place when a person is admitted to hospital with an illness such as an opportunistic infection or a disease such as tuberculosis that is AIDS-related. The processes of counselling described above – including breaking the news – should take place as part of the general patient care.

Treatment for AIDS patients involves treating the opportunistic infections, tuberculosis and troublesome and persistent symptoms such as diarrhoea, cough and itching (for more details of treatment see Chapter 3). Once a particular infection is treated a patient may appear to get better but the underlying immune deficiency is still present. They can maintain the quality of their lives and slow down the progress of the disease by *living positively* – eating well, avoiding exposure to other infections, taking adequate rest and leading as normal and rich a life as possible.

As discussed in Chapter 3 the emergence of combination therapy makes it now possible to substantially improve the quality of life of persons with AIDS. At present the high cost and need for trained health care staff has limited the use of combination therapy in most developing countries. Hopefully this situation will improve and combination therapy will become available as part of the routine treatment of all AIDS patients.

People with AIDS will also need to be counselled about avoiding the spread of HIV to others through sexual intercourse and be provided with condoms.

Counselling of the AIDS patient should be followed up by counselling of the family. The most important advice is to reassure family members and friends that HIV is not spread though normal social contact, bed linen and sharing of utensils. They should be advised to take simple measures to prevent spread of HIV and other infections.

Families of AIDS patients may need counselling if they are afraid that they have contracted HIV. With the spouse and sexual partner(s) of an AIDS patient you will need to discuss the possibility that they have also become infected with HIV. You can discuss the question of whether they should have a test for HIV. You should explain to them the importance of using condoms in their future sexual relations with the AIDS patient (or other persons).

Hospital- and home-based care of persons with AIDS

In 1989, WHO developed a broad definition of care as a 'comprehensive, integrated process which recognizes the range of needs for well being; it includes services and activities providing counselling and psycho-social support, nursing and medical care, legal, financial and practical services.'

There are different approaches for care of AIDS patients. Some hospitals keep them in ordinary wards whereas others have set up special wards for AIDS patients. As you saw in Chapters 3 and 4, HIV is not infectious in the hospital setting provided normal routine procedures of cleanliness are observed. Overreacting to the presence of AIDS patients by isolation and unnecessary sterile procedures will only increase the myths and fears about AIDS and reinforce the feeling of social isolation that AIDS patients feel. Other hospitals feel that it is appropriate to set up special wards. They argue that separation can protect the AIDS patient from other infectious diseases in the hospital. It can also ensure access to health care staff who are properly trained to provide the necessary care, counselling and support both to the AIDS patient as well as his/her sexual partner and family.

Health planners are increasingly worried by the financial cost of providing services for AIDS patients and the impact this will have on overstretched health budgets. Experiments are in progress with a range of alternatives to hospital care including community care, home visiting schemes and self-help groups.

The stay in hospital can be kept to a minimum if support is provided to enable families to care for AIDS patients. Although for many countries the initial interest in home-based care has been as ways of saving money, the benefits extend well beyond that of cost-cutting. They can mobilise the considerable reservoir of caring and sympathy that exists within a community. Involving the community in the care of AIDS patients will brings disease out in the open and confronts the myths and prejudices that surround it. Some of the needs that home-care services have to meet include:

- **Health care:** treatment of opportunistic diseases, TB, mental health, family planning.
- **Counselling and psychosocial support:** for the individual and family.
- **Advice on family and self care:** e.g. for diarrhoea, disposal or sterilisation of soiled materials, prevention of sexual transmission.
- **Economic support:** especially both income and food.
- **Support for children:** school fees, uniforms, child care.
- **Practical help in the home:** clothing, bedding, bandages, soap.
- **Legal help:** to prevent discrimination, to make a will.

The Chikankata Salvation Army Hospital in Zambia provides a good example of a rural home-based care programme set up in response to local needs in a rural community. The home-based care team consists of people from the AIDS care unit and visits the homes regularly. The objectives of the home visits are to assess the needs of those who are ill in a physical sense and to meet those needs through practical measures such as medicines and blankets. A secondary objective of the programme is to assess the impact of the education and counselling that was provided when the patient was at the hospital and during the earlier home visits. A third objective is to trace and provide counselling to any person who may have had sexual relations with the AIDS patient and other infected persons.

The programme supported by the Ndola Catholic Diocese in the Zambia's Copperbelt provides a good example of how volunteers can be used to provide home-based care in an urban community. The programme mobilised 500 volunteers to visit the homes of persons with AIDS and provide basic care, counselling and social support, organise home-care clinics in communities served by local health workers, liaise with hospitals and health facilities. The volunteers also supervise TB patients taking their medicines under the DOTS system.

There are considerable benefits in encouraging self-help groups where people with AIDS can meet and provide help and mutual support. This breaks down the feeling of guilt and isolation that a person with AIDS can feel. People with AIDS ('PWAs') are a resource that can be drawn upon to supplement stretched health care resources. Involvement in self-help groups and caring for others can provide a purpose and meaning for life. An example of a self-help group is The AIDS Support Organization (TASO) in Uganda.

Rejection and isolation have been experienced by AIDS patients in virtually all countries. However, traditional family structures in Africa and other developing societies have shown themselves to be caring and supportive to persons suffering from AIDS. The aim of community-based services should be to support these traditional structures wherever possible. This can involve establishing self-help and community care projects involving people with AIDS.

As the numbers of people suffering from AIDS increase, families will be severely stretched to provide support and care. This problem is being tackled in many countries and creative solutions are being found. For example in Uganda informal groups of women have been set up – called 'Muno Mu Kabi' (meaning 'a friend in need'). These women agree to provide support to each other in the case of difficulties such as deaths in the family from AIDS.

An approach common in Europe and USA, and now appearing in some parts of Africa, is to provide terminal care through residential institutions called hospices. For example the Mashambanzou NGO in Zimbabwe has converted a hospital ward into a hospice to care for terminally ill, destitute patients with AIDS and other illnesses who could not be cared for at home. They have also set up a residential unit in a suburb of Harare where patients can be admitted for a few days along with a family 'care giver' who receives training on how to look after the AIDS patient. Their facilities provide basic medical care but avoid the formal setting of the hospital. Their aim is to allow people with AIDS to die with dignity in caring and supportive surroundings.

After death of the AIDS patient some follow-up may still be necessary. A bereaved sexual partner or spouse may need counselling and social, financial and legal help – especially if they have been stigmatised by neighbours. The surviving spouse, may be under pressure to remarry – if he or she has children and needs help to care for them. However, the spouse is likely to be infected with HIV and this could lead to further spread of infection. Legal, economic and social help should be provided to enable widowed men and women to look after their children so that any decision to remarry is based on genuine choice.

Refugees and displaced people are vulnerable groups whose needs are often neglected. An appropriate response to meeting their needs for HIV/AIDS care must take into account: their already difficult situation; separation from family; difficult economic condition; traumatic experiences fleeing from violence; and uncertain future.

The impact of AIDS on children and AIDS orphans

UNAIDS, WHO and UNICEF define AIDS orphans as children who have lost their mother to AIDS before reaching the age of 15 years. Using this definition, they estimate 13 million children to have been orphaned by 2001. When one or both parents have AIDS the well-being of the whole family, including the children will be affected by the social, economic and psychological consequences of illness. Orphans run greater risk of being malnourished as they do not have parents to look after them. In some countries AIDS is increasingly a reason for school drop-out. In the final stages of illness of their parents, older children may have to leave school and work at home or in paid employment to support the family. The home-care services described above will need to take into account the needs of children in the families of those affected by AIDS.

When one or both parents have died, it is necessary to ensure that the orphaned children are properly cared for. Some AIDS orphans will themselves be infected with HIV and develop AIDS. The needs of children orphaned by AIDS fall into the following broad categories:

- **Physical needs:** food, clothing including footwear, blankets, housing and education.
- **Emotional and psychological needs:** counselling, love and attention to provide a sense of security and deal with the trauma and grief of the loss of parents, relatives and possibly a brother or sister.
- **Health care needs:** general preventive health care including immunisation, oral rehydration therapy, child health services; also support and care for child infected with HIV.
- **Education needs:** support to attend school – and a supportive school environment that is free from prejudice and discrimination.
- **Human rights needs:** protection from discrimination because of their HIV status and active educational programmes in communities to challenge the stigma of AIDS.

Examples of programmes addressing these needs are provided in the 'Strategies of Hope Series' details of which are provided at the end of the book. WAMATA in Tanzania is a good example of an AIDS support organisation that is addressing the needs of children as part of its home-based care programme. It was started in 1989 in Dar es Salaam and now has branches in many regions of the country. Activities are funded by contributions from the local community and donations from abroad. WAMATA aims to provide people with AIDS and their families with home-based medical and nursing care, social and psychological support, and also material assistance. Examples of the practical help it provides to children include supplying powdered milk to toddlers, and meeting the cost of school fees and uniforms. WAMATA is also helping to set up income earning schemes among families affected by AIDS including tailoring, livestock and fishing projects.

In Masvingo Province, Zimbabwe, the traditional structure of authority based on chiefs, was used as the basis for their programme of community-based care for orphans. With support of the chiefs, village development committees established local responses, which included gathering information on the extent of the problem of AIDS orphans, mobilising funds and building up a network of volunteers to ensure that orphans are properly fed, clothed, housed and stay in school.

The traditional pattern for caring for orphans in many societies is for the children to be taken into the families of relatives. However, as the AIDS epidemic develops, families can find it increasingly difficult to take in orphans unless help is provided. In some cultures there is no tradition of adoption and public education is needed to change attitudes about adoption. It is always better for a child to be looked after within a family. Unfortunately this is not always possible and care in an institution or orphanage may be necessary.

Many countries have set up national orphans programmes. Details of the AIDS orphan policy adopted by the Zimbabwe government were provided in the previous chapter (page 75). A national Orphan Programme was established in 1999 in Botswana which is run by various government departments, NGOs and community-based organisations. The programme is responsible for coordinating the registration of orphan data through a national database, identifying and addressing the needs of foster children and foster parents, training community volunteers in basic childcare, providing HIV/AIDS counselling and reviewing and developing government and child protection policies.

By the end of 1997, 6% of children under the age of 15 in Malawi were orphans. In response to the growing problem, Malawi's National Orphan Care Task Force had formed in 1992 and had developed the sub-region's first guidelines for the care of orphans which included:

- The first line of approach in orphan care must be in community-based programmes.
- Formal foster care will be expanded as the second most preferred type of care.
- Institutional care should be the last resort, through temporary care may be required for children awaiting placement.
- Hospitals should record next of kin so that relatives can be traced if children are abandoned.
- The registration of births and deaths should be improved to assist the monitoring of orphans.
- The Government will protect the property rights of orphans and these rights should be widely publicised.

- Self-help groups should be developed to help affected families with counselling and other needs.
- NGOs are encouraged to set up programmes of community-based care.
- The needs of all orphans should be considered on an equal basis, regardless of the cause of death of the parent or parents or their gender or religion.

As part of public education programmes it is important to stress that many AIDS orphans are not infected with HIV and, with appropriate care and support, will grow up to lead a normal life. They should be helped to achieve their potential. They are a nation's future.

Organisation of counselling services

Every health worker, teacher, employer etc. has a counselling function as part of their daily contacts within their communities. However, most countries have had to set up specialist counselling services for AIDS and STDs. Many approaches have been taken according to the level of HIV and AIDS in the community and available health and social services.

Counselling can take up much time both in the initial meeting and in follow-up sessions. It can be difficult for health and other field staff to fit it in alongside an already busy work schedule and services. A valuable approach is to select non-medical persons from the community with the right personal qualities and provide a basic training in AIDS and counselling. The best counsellor is not necessarily the one with the most education. Personal qualities such as understanding, patience and ability to express sympathy are essential. People generally respond better to a person of similar background and this needs to be considered when selecting counsellors for a particular group such as young people, older persons, men, women or sex workers.

An approach used by the Terence Higgins Trust in London is the *buddy* system. A volunteer is provided with some training and then given the responsibility of supporting a person with AIDS. This involves regularly visiting the AIDS patient at hospital or at home and being available at any time of the day to provide emotional support.

Persons who are HIV antibody positive have been found to make good counsellors. They have experienced themselves the shock of being diagnosed as HIV antibody positive and have had to come to terms with their situation.

Counselling service can be based on health facilities and be part of the process of testing, diagnosis and treatment. This can be complemented by 'drop-in' centres in easily accessible locations where people can come for help and advice and can be referred for testing if appropriate. These centres are often staffed by non-medical persons, volunteers and persons with AIDS. They may also provide a telephone counselling service or AIDS 'hot-line'. Counselling programmes often combine counselling with general AIDS education activities in the community. An approach used in one programme in Africa was for the counsellors to see clients in the mornings and go into the community to do AIDS education in the afternoon.

Volunteers are an important component of many of the programmes described above. In some programmes the motivation to volunteer has come from religious beliefs and a desire to serve the community. In other programmes incentives may be given to volunteers such as subsidised food and transport. Being a volunteer is very demanding both in time and emotions. It is important to be realistic about how much you can expect a volunteer can do. If they are to function properly, volunteers need support from health and other services, their families/partners and the community – even more so if the volunteers themselves are HIV positive and have their own need for support.

Whoever becomes involved in counselling, they should receive training on the specific communication/counselling/caring skills needed for fulfilling their role. Counselling and caring for people with HIV and AIDS is demanding and stressful. Counsellors can easily 'burn-out' under the strain and their training should help prepare them for this. Follow-up should be provided to enable counsellors to share experiences and create mutual support networks.

Role play is a method that is widely used in training and is shown in Figure 10. Difficult situations can be acted out and participants can practise giving advice and discussing different approaches.

This chapter has provided examples of some of the issues and approaches in meeting the needs of persons with HIV/AIDS. The experiences of home care and self-help projects have been described in publications of UNAIDS and the excellent series of publications in the 'Strategies of Hope' series that are listed at the end of this book. One of the challenges is to find ways of scaling up these small projects without losing the commitment and energy that have made them so successful. This will involve the coordination and mobilisation of government agencies such as health and social services, NGOs including churches, industry and community groups. All have a vital role to play.

7. An action plan for fighting AIDS

With accessible vaccines or treatment still only a distant prospect for most of the developing world, the AIDS epidemic can only be controlled through a massive programme involving action at the individual, family, community, national and global level. The key to success is communication, which in its many different forms is the focus of this chapter. Communication can involve two main kinds of activities: education and advocacy.

Advocacy is the process by which individuals and groups try to influence local and national leaders, policy makers and the media to change laws and adopt policies that will control AIDS (such as development of an effective AIDS control programme), provide appropriate health/counselling services, protect human rights and address underlying economic and social issues.

Educational programmes are activities directed at whole communities or targeted at specific individuals and groups. They seek to provide information, influence beliefs and attitudes, counter stigma and prejudice, provide decision-making skills and empower people to change themselves and their community.

Each of us can contribute to the fight against AIDS in different ways. Through our:

- **Professional roles**, e.g. as health workers, teachers, employers, trade unionists, church ministers, politicians, social workers, media journalists, police.
- **Community roles** through our social contacts with others in the community and workplace and through participation in social, religious and political structures.
- **Family role** as family members and parents.

This chapter will describe how you can develop a programme of AIDS education in your community and suggest guidelines for effective communication. In the space available it is only possible to concentrate on the main principles of effective education applied to

AIDS and STDs. You can find a detailed discussion of health education in my book *Communicating Health – an action guide to health education and health promotion –* also published by Macmillan.

Guidelines for effective educational programmes

Encouraging a teamwork approach
It is easy to become discouraged by the task of changing such well-established and sensitive sexual behaviours on the scale that is needed to control the AIDS epidemic. This can only be done if everyone works together. You can see below examples of groups that can be mobilised at the community level to form an action group or committee to promote AIDS education in your community.

Groups that can be mobilised

Voluntary agencies:
  voluntary health associations
  Red Cross/Red Crescent Societies
  family planning associations

Government agencies:
  health workers
  teachers
  adult educators
  social workers
  youth workers
  community development workers
  agricultural extension

Media journalists:
  newspapers
  radio
  television

Individuals/groups:
  religious leaders
  trade unionists
  women's organisations
  community leaders
  traditional healers
  boy scouts/girl guides
  village committees
  bar keepers

Choosing target groups

Although everyone is at risk – each section of the public will have different needs. A comprehensive AIDS prevention programme will direct health education at a range of different groups with education approaches specific for each. Possible target groups could include:

- parents and school children,
- young persons,
- married couples – husbands and wives,
- men and women working away from home,
- sex workers (prostitutes),

- patients at STD clinics,
- injecting drug users,
- men who have sex with men (homosexual men),
- prisoners,
- police, soldiers, sailors,
- professional groups, e.g. health workers/teachers,
- traditional healers,
- religious and community leaders/elders/politicians,
- employers and trade unions,
- journalists.

The term *primary target group* is used for the people whose sexual behaviour you wish to influence. *Secondary target groups* are persons that you wish to reach because of the influence that they can have on others, e.g. the parent over the child, the mother-in-law over the daughters-in-law, the husband over the wife.

Involving the community

You should involve as many different groups as possible in your health education. Can you find out who are the respected people with influence in your community? Spend time talking to them and find out what they think about AIDS and the safer sex message. Invite them to participate in planning and carrying out health education activities.

Increasing recognition is being made of the value of involving HIV antibody positive persons and people with AIDS. They can contribute through mutual self-help and sharing with others their feelings and needs. In TASO (The AIDS Support Organisation) in Uganda, persons who are HIV antibody positive give support to each other. This tackles the stigma and prejudice surrounding AIDS by bringing it out into the open.

Another group who have been involved in many countries are sex workers (prostitutes); they are in a good position to advise on the best way of reaching other sex workers in their community.

This 'community-based' or 'out-reach' approach has already been successful in family planning programmes and has considerable potential for AIDS control. It ensures that educational messages are relevant and effective. Usually people are more easily reached and convinced by a trusted member of their own group than by an outsider. Involving others will increase the effectiveness of your own work. Another name for this approach is 'peer education'.

Learning about your community

If you are going to communicate effectively you will need to learn about your audience. What do they already know and feel about AIDS, STDs, condoms and the safer-sex behaviours? Do they think that AIDS can be prevented? Can they recognise the symptoms of sexually transmitted diseases? Do they think that they are at risk? What additional information do they want to know about AIDS?

It is important to know the local myths and customs that may affect the spread of AIDS and STDs. Can you identify any incorrect beliefs that you will have to try to change? With the expansion of public education programmes, most people now accept that AIDS is sexually transmitted. However, in many countries there is still confusion about modes of transmission. Many people still believe that AIDS can be transmitted by donating one's blood, insect bites and casual contact. These misunderstandings are dangerous because they encourage people to practise harmful behaviours or avoid safe behaviours such as giving blood. Misunderstandings about the low risk of HIV infection from casual contact can also lead to fear and discrimination against persons who are diagnosed with AIDS or who are HIV antibody positive.

Not all traditional beliefs are obstacles. Many emphasise family values such as faithfulness and caring for sick members of the family. Can you identify local beneficial beliefs that you can reinforce and build upon?

Where research has already been carried out, the results can guide you on what messages need to be reinforced. However, it is not always necessary to do large scale surveys of Knowledge, Attitudes, Beliefs and Practice ('KABP'). Discussions with individuals and small groups of people can provide much information about attitudes and beliefs. A good way to find out relevant information is to see what people think about the AIDS education materials that have already been produced and whether they agree with the information presented.

Choosing appropriate messages

From our discussions in earlier chapters on the transmission and prevention of HIV and AIDS the following points might be relevant to include in your education:

- AIDS is a fatal disease, there is no cure.
- It is transmitted only through sex, blood and from mother to children; it is not transmitted through casual contact or insects.
- Once infected, it can take from 2 to 10 years or even longer to develop the disease; during that period a person shows no

symptoms but can infect others.

- Persons with AIDS and HIV should be treated with compassion and their rights must be respected. Everyone is at risk of HIV and they should not be blamed or victimised for their misfortune.
- It is impossible to tell by appearance who is infected with the virus; you must assume that anyone with whom you have intercourse is infected unless you are really sure of that person.
- Everyone is at risk of becoming infected if they do not take these sensible precautions:
  - Young people should delay having sexual intercourse until they are ready to embark on a regular relationship.
  - Reduce the number of sexual partners; ideally stick to one regular sexual partner; avoid sex with people who have many sex partners.
  - Practise low risk forms of sexual intercourse (listed earlier).
  - If you develop symptoms of sexually transmitted diseases such as abnormal discharges from the penis or vagina, sores in the genital area or pain during urination, go to a clinic for treatment.
  - Only use health services and traditional healers who sterilise their instruments.
- Say no to drugs! Drugs can harm your health and destroy your mind. They could even kill you.
  - Don't inject drugs. It's less dangerous to take drugs by mouth or inhalation.
  - If you are using drugs – get help to give up.
  - Sharing needles can spread diseases like AIDS. If you inject drugs either use a new disposable syringe each time or sterilise your syringe in bleach. Never share your syringe and needles with others.

These points will need to be adapted to the culture and needs of your own community. You should resist pressure to adopt unrealistic messages such as 'one sexual partner for life'. This is far removed from the current state of sexual activity in many communities – basing a health education programme on it will be ineffective and lead to people laughing at you and not taking you seriously. Do not pass moral judgements on the sexual activities of the communities you work with and concentrate on making existing sexual practices safe through adopting low-risk behaviours and use of condoms.

It is essential at the beginning of your health education work to avoid the problem of conflicting and confusing messages. You should meet politicians, local leaders, parents, health workers, journalists and other media persons to discuss the moral issues and agree on acceptable and effective messages.

Your community may find it difficult to understand many of the facts about HIV-related diseases given in earlier chapters of this book. Many people are not aware of the existence of the immune system. It is difficult to explain to them that HIV infects and damages the immune system. People may also find it hard to understand the concept of opportunistic infections and why patients with different illnesses, such as diarrhoea, tuberculosis or shingles are all diagnosed as AIDS.

There is widespread confusion about the difference between having full symptoms of the disease AIDS and the carrier HIV antibody positive state where a person shows no symptoms but can still infect others. This is an important distinction that you will have to emphasise repeatedly. Another point to emphasise is the long incubation period. You should explain: that the cases appearing now may have been infected up to 10 years ago; and there will be many more symptom-free carriers, showing no symptoms, capable of infecting others who are likely to develop AIDS. However, you need to be sensitive to your audience. Almost certainly some of them will be HIV antibody positive. Your educational activities could increase the stress and anxiety they may already feel.

How to put across your message

You do not have to go into complex details of viruses, the immune system and the pathology of the disease in order to justify the safer-sex message. Build on ideas of health, disease and family values that the community already has. For example in Kenya the slogan 'zero grazing' has been adopted. This is a concept used by cattle herdsmen to describe the practice of keeping a cow tied to a stake so it only grazes in a single place and doesn't wander!

In communities where there have been few AIDS cases the issue can seem remote and abstract. The challenge is to make it seem real and important, but at the same time keeping it in context with the other concerns and problems that people are facing. A sensible approach is to make sure that health education on AIDS also refers to sexually transmitted diseases that people will already know something about.

Do not try to frighten your community into action. It's unfortunate that some of the early posters produced showed skeletons and skulls. People can respond to frightening messages by laughing them off and denying them. Even worse you may add to the panic and fear surrounding AIDS when your message should be one of reassurance that the disease can be prevented. You should always include a clear statement on what actions your audience can take to reduce their risk of AIDS and where they can go for advice.

Humour is sometimes helpful in discussion of serious topics as it can lighten the tension. Simple emotional approaches showing the importance of caring relationships can also have strong appeal.

People want to enjoy life and can resent messages using words such as 'avoid ...' and 'don't ...'. Be positive in your advice and tell people what they *can* do. Show safer sex as something worthwhile, exciting and pleasurable rather than an inferior version of ordinary sex. Put over your health education in an entertaining way to attract interest and hold attention. Only use medical information and technical terms if you are sure that the audience has the education to understand them.

Use the local expressions and slang for words such as sexual intercourse, oral sex, anal intercourse, penis, semen, vagina. For example in some parts of Africa condoms are called gumboots and raincoats! The technical terms and the polite expressions that we often use may save embarrassment but can make the health education distant and remote. Using everyday expressions helps to build a bridge between you and the community.

Whatever appeal or message you use, it is essential that you *pre-test* them. Show drafts of your posters, leaflets, radio programmes or other media to samples from your intended audience. Make sure that your messages are understood, that people do not react strongly against them and that you do not unwittingly contribute to the stigma of AIDS in the way the message is presented. Some different appeals are shown in Figure 12. Look at these and think which attracts you most and which you think are more suited for AIDS education.

Planning educational programmes in the community

Reaching women

Women have their distinct needs and some of these have already been discussed in previous chapter. In many societies women have less access to education, including information about many health topics including AIDS and STDs. The stigma attached to having an STD may mean that, even if they recognise that they are infected, women can be reluctant to seek treatment from a health worker. Furthermore their weak economic position often forces them to be dependent on men for support which can make it difficult for them to insist on safer sex.

Another area of increasing concern in some African and Middle East countries is female circumcision – now called 'female genital mutilation'.

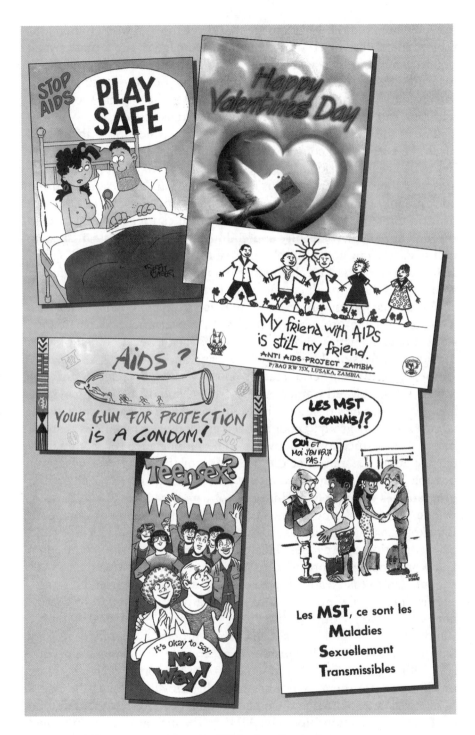

Figure 12. Different appeals used in AIDS education leaflets

It is now believed that the damage that this causes to women increases their vulnerability to HIV transmission. Damage to the female sexual organs can also be caused by other practices designed to enhance male pleasure during intercourse such as drying out the vagina before intercourse or treatment with herbs to tighten the vagina. Violent sex and rape can also increase the risk of HIV transmission.

One of the early lessons learned from AIDS education is that AIDS has to be seen in the context of other problems women face. Support has to be given, and skills developed, so that women can negotiate safer sex with their partners and insist on protection. This requires using educational methods that not only give facts and demonstrate how to use condoms but *empower* women to act. You can reach many women through antenatal, maternity and child health clinics. You can arrange group discussions and counselling sessions to explain AIDS and STDs. However, this will not reach younger women before their first pregnancy who will not have much contact with health services.

You can also set up programmes to reach women in their workplaces. This is possible in large factories or government departments. Educational activities should be directed at all levels of employees including professional, secretarial, catering and cleaning staff.

You will find it harder to reach women working in small factories or offices, self-employed women such as traders and women living in rural areas. Women's organisations, including market traders' organisations, adult education groups, cooperatives and other associations, can be involved in educational activities. The importance of community participation was raised at the beginning of this chapter – whenever possible, decisions on the content and running of AIDS education programmes should be put into the control of women themselves.

The 'Empower' programme among the 4000 women bar workers in Bangkok, Thailand, provides an example of the use of participatory and peer education approaches. Health education, bar visits, counselling and workshops were provided to 4000 women bar workers who were encouraged to take leadership roles in educating their friends.

It is often totally unrealistic to expect a married woman to change her sexual behaviour without her husband's approval. Double standards exist: while it is considered proper for women to stay faithful, many men still consider it acceptable to have extra-marital sex. Although women may not object to condoms, men are often unwilling to use them. AIDS has brought into sharp focus the issues of relative status of men and women and the need for trust and mutual confidence in relationships. The AIDS epidemic cannot be controlled without improvements in the status of women.

Reaching men

There are groups of men that are at special risk of HIV infection. When men are away from their home and families there is increased likelihood of casual sex and use of sex workers. Such men at risk can include those who have travelled to the cities for work or even to another country as migrant labourers. A vulnerable situation is provided whenever men are grouped together such as in the army, navy, merchant navy, hostels and prisons.

Can you take health education to where men are? This means developing educational programmes within workplaces (discussed later in this chapter), in churches and mosques and being prepared to go out at night to people's homes and bars and dance halls. Can you use men as fieldworkers? They can be trained to talk frankly using everyday language about sexual matters.

Men at special risk both for catching and spreading AIDS are long distance drivers who have sex with women at stops along the highways. In Tanzania an AIDS education project was set up at seven truck stops along the TanZam Highway. A starting point was to identify all bars, guesthouse, pombe (locally brewed beer) shops, disco halls and truck stands. The programme then went on to train female bar workers and male petrol station attendants as peer educators. They worked as volunteers giving AIDS education and distributing condoms to truck drivers, barmaids and other groups. As a result of the programme, condoms have become more acceptable. Truck drivers started to put the white condom boxes by their windscreen 'to assure barmaids that we constantly use condoms and are therefore safe. It attracts them.' (!!)

Because they are often travelling, truck drivers can delay going to clinics if they have an STD. In Mombasa, Kenya, mobile health clinics were held one morning each week in the depots of each of six of the largest trucking companies. As well as treating infections, informal group discussions were held. In India another approach was to set up free roadside tea houses with STD clinics.

Truck driver programmes have been set up by national AIDS programmes, e.g. in Malawi; by NGOs, e.g. STOPAIDS in Nigeria; and employers, e.g. the Zimbabwe National Employment Council for the Transport Operating Industry. A problem encountered with some of these programmes is that, while success has been achieved in getting drivers to use condoms with sex workers, it has been more difficult to get them to use condoms with their regular partners.

There are many examples of successful programmes with men who have sex with men in the Americas, Europe and Australia. Increasingly programmes are being set up in countries where homosexuality was not recognised previously, e.g. in Asia. Carrying out educational work with gays is difficult in countries where there is no organised gay movement to act as a focus for community involvement. For example, health education workers in Beijing, China, have had to make regular visits to public parks and other meeting places to make contact and win the confidence of men and provide confidential help through a telephone hotline. It is also difficult when legal, religious and social sanctions drive homosexuality underground. Human rights, the law and the prevention of AIDS are all linked.

While important, finding new and imaginative ways of reaching men is not the only answer. In AIDS programmes men have often been portrayed as the villains oppressing women. Increasingly it is realised that men themselves are also victims of male stereotypes. Educational programmes need to consider the deeper values and ideas in society that contribute to unsafe sex by men especially that of machismo and sexual prowess. One of the challenges is to find alternative forms of expression of masculinity which build on positive attributes of 'maleness' but are consistent with responsibility, caring for others and safer sex. These alternative values can only be developed with the full participation of men themselves in the search for solutions.

AIDS education in the workplace

The importance of the workplace as a way of reaching both men and women has already been discussed in previous sections. As the AIDS epidemic develops, there has been increased awareness of the economic consequences of AIDS in lost productivity, drain on skilled workers and human suffering. In some work situations there may be an additional risk of infection with HIV where there is contact with blood, e.g. hospital work. Another source of risk comes from sexual harassment where women may be under pressure from employers to have sex.

The book *Work Against AIDS* in the 'Strategies of Hope' series, gives examples of many workplace initiatives in Zimbabwe. These include AIDS education activities in textile factories, commercial farms, tea estates, mining companies. For one company, the David Whitehead Textile Company, the trigger to act was the discovery that almost one quarter (22%) of blood donors from two factories were HIV antibody positive. These programmes used a peer education approach and trained workers to carry out education to others. This resulted in an increased level of condom utilisation and a visible impact of their efforts has been a decline in STDs.

The Zimbabwe experience emphasised the importance of obtaining the commitment of both the management and workforce, including trade unions, in an educational programme that is sustained over time and supported by a *Workplace AIDS Policy*, distribution of condoms and accessible facilities for health care, including STD treatment.

Employers and trade unions in many other countries have cooperated to develop AIDS policies for their workplaces. These policies typically include actions to prevent discrimination against recruitment of HIV antibody positive persons, safeguards to protect infected workers and AIDS education and counselling of the workforce. In 1990 the World Health Organization, International Labour Office and League of Red Cross and Red Crescent Societies produced the following guidelines on HIV/AIDS in the workplace.

Extracts from WHO/ILO Guidelines on HIV/AIDS and the Workplace

PERSONS IN EMPLOYMENT
1. **HIV/AIDS screening:** HIV/AIDS screening, whether direct, indirect or asking questions about tests already taken, should not be required.
2. **Confidentiality:** Confidentiality regarding all medical information including HIV/AIDS status, must be maintained.
3. **Informing the employer:** There should be no obligation for the employee to inform the employer regarding his or her HIV/AIDS status.
4. **Protection of employee:** Persons in the workplace affected by, or perceived to be affected by HIV/AIDS, must be protected from stigmatization and discrimination by co-workers, unions, employers or clients. Information and education are essential to maintain the climate of mutual understanding necessary to ensure this protection.
5. **Access to services:** Employees and their families should have access to information and educational programmes on HIV/AIDS as well as to appropriate referral.
6. **Benefits:** HIV-infected employees should not be discriminated against, and should have access to standard social security benefits and occupationally related benefits.
7. **Reasonable changes in working arrangements:** HIV infection by itself is not associated with any limitation in fitness to work. If fitness to work is impaired by HIV-related illness, reasonable alternative working arrangements should be made.
8. **Continuation of employment:** HIV infection is not a cause for termination of employment. As with many other illnesses, persons with HIV-related illnesses should be able to work as long as medically fit for available appropriate work.
9. **First aid:** In any situation requiring first aid in the workplace, precautions need to be taken to reduce the risk of transmitting blood-borne infections, including hepatitis B. These standard precautions will be equally effective against HIV transmission.

In 1997, the 14 member states of the Southern African Development Community (SADC) agreed on a *Code of Best Practice around AIDS and Employment* which built upon and expanded these guidelines.

AIDS education through places of worship

Religious institutions such as churches and mosques provide a valuable way of involving communities in AIDS control. There are many examples of successful involvement of religious groups. The Islamic Medical Association of Uganda, formed in 1988 has provided training for Imams on AIDS, established dialogue between Islamic leaders and health services and initiated community health education activities. Christian mission hospitals such as Chikenkata Hospital in Zambia have carried out pioneering work on home care. Religious institutions are able to mobilise large sections of the community and address the many difficult spiritual and moral issues involved in AIDS education.

Reaching young people at school and college

It is important to carry out health education with school children. Young children are a section of the community who are normally free from HIV and it is important to ensure that they do not become infected. In Uganda, this period of life normally free from infection has been called the 'Window of opportunity'. However, this window does not stay open for long. Many children begin experimenting with sex while still at school. Later, away from home at college, they will be exposed to many temptations. School girls are often enticed to have sex with older men or 'sugar daddies' in exchange for money or gifts.

Children can learn about AIDS from sessions in the classroom. But they also learn a great deal from the 'hidden curriculum' that the school provides through the personal example of the teachers, the climate of relationships in the school including rewards and punishment. This may be at a general level or at a specific level in the school's response to AIDS and HIV. For example, many schools have had to face the situation where one of their pupils or a teacher has been infected with HIV through sex, blood transfusion or contaminated blood products. There is very little risk of infection of others through casual contact, yet in the early days of the AIDS epidemic fears and misunderstandings led parents to threaten to withdraw their children when they heard that a child or teacher was infected with HIV. If parents, pupils and teachers respond that way, the myths, misconceptions and stigma that surround AIDS will be reinforced in children's minds.

Some important decisions must be taken which include: when to introduce the topics AIDS and sexually transmitted diseases to children; where in the syllabus it should be included; and who should teach it? It is tempting to leave teaching about AIDS and sexually transmitted diseases until children are over 14 years old or in secondary school. This is too late as some pupils will have already started sexual activities. UNAIDS reported on a survey of 1600 children in a poor area of Lusaka, Zambia. Over a quarter of children aged 10 said that they already had had sex and the figure rose to 60% among 14 year olds. In South Africa 10% of a sample had started having sex from the age of 11 years. In a survey of teenage girls in Kisumu, Kenya, one girl in 10 was infected by her 15th birthday. Education on AIDS and sexual behaviour should start as early as possible.

It is best if education on AIDS is not treated separately but is carried out as part of a general health education programme including other sexually transmitted diseases and personal relationships. This should begin in the primary school with basic concepts of health and disease as well as human relationships and then progress to more detailed treatment as children get older. Increasing attention is being placed in using a 'life skills' approach which emphasises activity-based learning methods that allow pupils to discover issues for themselves and practice decision-making skills. Good examples of these are seen in the activity sheets freely available from the Child-to-Child Programme.

There may be parts of the existing syllabus called 'health education' where the topics of AIDS and sexually transmitted diseases can be included. However, it is also possible to deal with these topics and explore relationships, feelings and prejudices in an effective way in subjects such as biology, religious studies, English, drama, music and out of school activities. For example in Zambia Anti-AIDS clubs have been set up where pupils meet after school to discuss AIDS and its implications on their lives.

Outside health workers can play a useful role but the teachers themselves should take responsibility for the AIDS education in the school. They are in the school all the time and can provide guidance and counselling to students with special problems. However, teachers will need support and training to help them deal with the many difficult issues raised when discussing AIDS and sexuality in the classroom. You will also have to be realistic in the expectations you

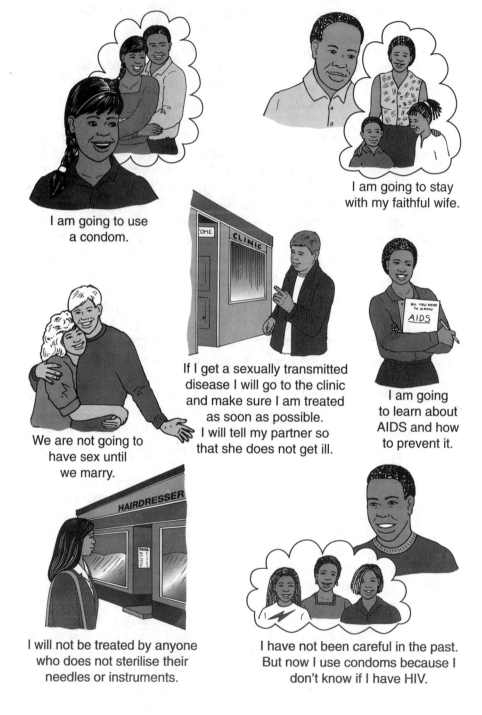

Figure 13. Samples of school health education from the Living Health Series

place on teachers who are often working under difficult conditions with overcrowded classrooms and shortages – and in many cases a total absence – of books and other teaching materials. The personal needs of teachers will also have to met in any training as they themselves are members of society and at risk from AIDS. It has been estimated that in the first 10 months of 1998 in Zambia 1300 teachers died from AIDS – equivalent to two-thirds of the annual output of the teacher training colleges during that same year.

In the past some parents have objected to sex education in schools. Now, because of AIDS, they are increasingly willing to allow sex education in schools. It's a good idea to hold a meeting with teachers and parents and discuss what you wish to do and involve them. In this way the parents will reinforce the AIDS education given at school. AIDS education programmes in many countries have begun to develop curricula for sexually transmitted diseases and AIDS as well as to train teachers to teach this sensitive area.

Many parents are concerned that informing young people about safer sex, including condoms, is likely to encourage them to experiment with sex. There is no evidence to suggest that this occurs. We must remember that young people will already know something about sex but that their information is likely to be wrong or incomplete. It is far better that they should get correct information from a responsible adult rather than rely on gossip from friends. Furthermore, studies reviewed by UNAIDS as part of their 'Best Practice' series have shown that sex education does not encourage promiscuity. Instead it can help young people make sensible decisions such as delaying the onset of sexual activity and taking the necessary precautions to avoid pregnancy and STDs.

Students at technical colleges, teachers in training colleges and universities are another important group. They are often away from home for the first time and beginning to become sexually active. As potential leaders of the future they are a high priority group in which to minimise the risk of AIDS, as well as being in a position to influence others in the community. AIDS education programmes in colleges involve running education sessions with students, strengthening counselling services and establishing guidelines to preserve the rights of HIV infected pupils.

Reaching young people out of school

Out-of-school children include the following groups: school children in their spare time; children who have left school early and are now working; and children who have never gone to school at all – these could be children orphaned by wars and disease or deserted by their parents through poverty or whose parents have died of AIDS. Also important are the growing numbers of *street children* in cities of Latin America, Africa and Asia who earn money from petty trading, parking cars, and in some situations theft and child prostitution. In Lusaka in Zambia in 1991 there were some 35,000 children living on the streets. Ten years later that number had more than doubled to around 75,000. Many of these out-of-school children will AIDS orphans. A review by UNICEF in 1999 describes alarming survey data from Zambia which showed that 32% of the orphans in urban Lusaka and a shocking 68% in rural areas were not receiving schooling

School health education programmes can miss those children who do not progress to secondary school or who drop out. There is a gender gap with girls forming more than 60% of the drop-outs because of the low priority placed on education of women in many communities. When they leave school, young people become more independent from their parents and begin to earn some money. They are more likely to be sexually active than school children at the same age. They are also likely to have been the victims of economic and sexual exploitation.

Young people out of school are one of the most difficult groups to reach. If they attend youth clubs, educational activities can be carried out in these informal locations. However, many young people do not attend them and imaginative approaches are needed to reach these groups. Could you use a more informal approach? Many young people want to be independent from their families and will resent being talked to like children. Indeed, one advantage of educational programmes outside the school is that it is possible to be much more informal and relaxed in advice than in the school or family setting.

Some promising approaches that have been used for working with young people are to:

- Use people that young people look up to such as singers or football players to speak on health issues.
- Ask popular music groups to perform songs about health issues.
- Use young people as fieldworkers that youths will listen and respond to.
- Involve young people themselves in producing a drama about their lives and situation.
- Use a 'peer education' approach, e.g. train a group of young volunteers to carry out informal health education in the bars and discos where the young people go.

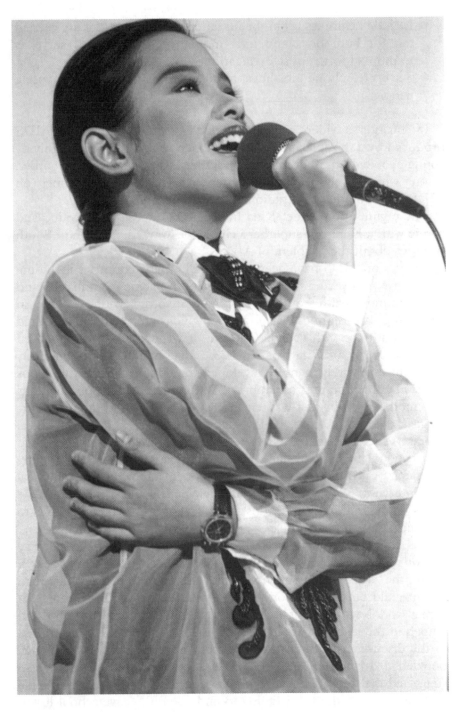

Figure 14. Using music to reach young people – Lea Salonga in the Philippines
(Credit: John Harris)

- Include health issues in the initiation ceremonies that are carried out for both boys and girls in many countries and serve as traditional forms of sex education.
- Set up telephone 'hot-lines' to give confidential advice to young people.

In Uganda a video was made of a song and drama on AIDS produced by a musician who was looked up to and regarded highly by young people. Remo Fernandes, a popular Indian singer, has recorded a song with a lively beat called 'Safer sex'. In Malawi 'rap songs' on AIDS were broadcast on radio and distributed on cassette.

The organisation Street Kids International developed a video and comic with a Kung Fu superhero character to warn children in South America about the problem of AIDS.

Comics on AIDS have been produced in many countries including Zimbabwe, Kenya and the Pacific. The South Pacific Commission and the Commonwealth Youth Programme involved young people in producing two comics *Pacific Wize* which are being distributed throughout the South Pacific. One country, Tonga, has even serialised the comic in its local newspaper. *Radical* is a highly popular monthly magazine for young people developed and published by the Athos Bulcâo Foundation in Brasilia, Brazil. With bright colours, photographs and modern layout and written in easy-to-understand language, the magazine covers cultural issues such as literature and music, social concerns such as human rights and politics, and personal matters such as sex and relationships. It takes an interactive approach, whereby young people are asked to contribute articles, poems and drawings. Radical also interviews young people about their beliefs and aspirations. One of its more radical innovations is to arrange for young people to interview government ministers, teachers, artists and musicians.

It is important to involve young people themselves. The Zimbabwe National Family Planning Council (ZNFPC) consulted young people about the issues that were important to them. The youth named parent-child communication, dealing with 'sugar daddies', choice of career and boy-girl relationships. Some of the teenagers who had helped in the research wrote their own stories about the issues raised in the discussions – this led to the story now included in a 20-page booklet in cartoon style called 'Facts about growing up'. They also suggested the words for a song about sugar daddies 'Don't go boogie with old men ... the fun is going to end ... you'll leave school if you boogie with old men ... he will desert you ... alone pushing along with the pregnancy ... what will you support the baby with?'

The Philippine young people's project used an enter-educate strategy which involved a multi-media campaign centred around two 'pop' songs and music videos with messages about sexual responsibility and prevention of teenage pregnancy. These coincided with the launching of a telephone hotline 'Dial-a-friend'. A singer, Lea Salonga, was teamed up with a group to produce the songs and commercial sponsorship was also received for the project. Free television and air-time was given to play the records and for appearances of the group. Volunteer counsellors were trained for the telephone hotline which was also promoted through TV and radio spots

The peer education approach of training young volunteers to carry out health education to other young people has been used successfully in many countries. Young people are strongly influenced by their friends ('peers') and fashions; this source of pressure can be made use of in your health education. In, the largest slum area of Nairobi, the Mathare Youth Sports Association has been training its footballers to be peer educators about HIV. Members of the senior squad, were the first to be trained. They stress abstinence from sex; but for those who are sexually active, they emphasise the importance of using condoms and staying faithful to one partner.

These educational approaches will have to be combined with practical measures such as job training, employment generation and protection from harassment if there is to be any meaningful impact on street children.

Sex workers

The sex worker is both at risk of becoming infected with AIDS and of spreading it to others. Injecting drug users sometimes turn to sex work to finance their addiction.

Sex workers can be women, men or transvestites (men dressed as women) and even children. In recent years there has been a rise in 'sex tourism' where the availability of female and male sex workers is part of the attraction of going to a particular country or resort.

The term 'prostitute' is not a helpful one as it covers a wide range of practices and arouses prejudices and strong feelings and leads to stigma. At one end of a spectrum are men and women who have sexual relationships in return for gifts and a good time out. Then there are those who have sex in exchange for cash on an occasional basis. At the other end of the spectrum are sex workers who can have as many as 1000 partners in a year.

Educational programmes have now been undertaken with sex workers in many countries in The Americas, Europe, Africa and Asia.

These programmes have involved providing regular health checks and treatment for any sexually transmitted diseases. When effort is made to explain the facts about AIDS, sex workers have been found to be willing to insist that their clients use condoms. An ingredient for success is that of providing counselling, group discussion and using peer education approaches that directly involves them in AIDS education among their fellow sex workers.

One of the first documented AIDS education programmes with sex workers was carried out in Nairobi, Kenya. In 1988 the programme reported the encouraging news that intensive health education could increase the use of condoms by female sex workers and their clients. The study also reported the finding that regular condom use reduced the risk of the female sex workers themselves becoming infected with HIV.

Since then, successful programmes with sex workers have been carried out in many countries. It is usually possible to identify and work with the full-time sex workers especially if they are based at well-defined locations such as brothels or bars or have their own associations. However, it is very difficult to contact women who meet their clients in the street or are only involved in sex work on an occasional basis. The legal status of sex work can also be an obstacle to the control of AIDS and STDs. It is difficult to develop effective educational programmes in countries where sex work is illegal and is driven 'underground'. Legal reforms were discussed as one of the strategies for prevention described in Chapter 5. In Europe, sex workers have formed an alliance to press for their rights.

A long-term perspective must consider the economic pressures that push women into sex work. Women are often forced into sex work through the need for money to maintain their families and children. So it is unrealistic to expect them to stop their work unless alternative sources of income are provided and AIDS control programmes are increasingly addressing this issue.

The issue of sex work is one where double standards exist, with a tendency to blame women rather than the men who use them! Many people feel that there has been too much focus on AIDS and STD control with sex workers. This has reinforced the stigma on these groups and also led other sections of the community to become complacent about their own risk. Clients of sex workers have been ignored by education and prevention projects. Educational programmes for sex workers should be part of a comprehensive educational strategy that which reaches out to all sections of the community.

AIDS education in prisons

Prisoners, both male and female, are a group whose needs for AIDS education have only recently been recognised. The level of HIV infection in prisons is often higher than among the general population. HIV can be transmitted within prisons by homosexual intercourse and drug injection. In the United States an official enquiry reported in September 1993 that AIDS was responsible for nearly 30% of all deaths in US prisons.

In 1993 the World Health Organization condemned compulsory testing of prisoners as 'unethical, ineffective and discriminatory'. UNAIDS has included guidelines on prisons and AIDS in its 'Best Practice' series which includes calls for distribution of condoms for prisoners, setting up of needle exchange programmes, the provision of confidential testing including pre- and post-test counselling, no isolation of prisoners on grounds of their HIV status, adequate measures to combat sexual violence including rape. The high level of TB among prisoners has already been discussed in Chapter 6. Screening for TB and treatment using the DOTS approach should be made available for all prisoners.

Imaginative health education approaches are needed to educate prisoners and prison staff. In Maputo, Mozambique, 30 prisoners were trained as peer educators. An evaluation programme showed that their health education led to an increase in knowledge about AIDS among the other prisoners.

Promoting condoms

You have already seen in an earlier chapter that the promotion of proper use of male and female condoms is an important part of programmes to reduce the incidence of sexually transmitted diseases and HIV. In some countries there has been a long tradition of condom promotion within family planning programmes. However, condoms have never been very popular as a contraceptive method and we have to understand the reasons why, in order to overcome these problems in future AIDS control programmes.

Surveys in the early 1980s showed a low level of use of condoms. The availability of the contraceptive pill as an extremely reliable and convenient method is one reason for this low use of condoms. Another reason has been the complaint among couples that it interferes with the spontaneity of love making and reduces pleasurable sensations. Men or women can be shy to ask shopkeepers for condoms. They may not want to be seen to be carrying condoms in case they are called promiscuous.

People are often reluctant to use a condom because they think it is inconvenient and will reduce the pleasure of lovemaking. In response to this criticism you can point out that using condoms is a question of establishing a different routine that can be just as pleasurable. Anxiety and uncertainty about the possibility of becoming infected with HIV and other sexually transmitted diseases can also spoil lovemaking and using a condom can remove that anxiety. People may have heard that condoms are unreliable and break. However, in an earlier chapter we showed that condoms can be very reliable if used properly. You will need to reassure them that if used properly condoms are very reliable. A good way of showing how strong they are is to blow one up to show how large a balloon it makes before bursting!

It's a good idea to look for men who use condoms regularly and are happy with them. You can ask these 'satisfied users' their reasons for using the condoms and how they use them. This can provide ideas that you can build into your health education programme. You can even use these persons as health educators to explain the use of condoms among persons in their workplace or community.

Do not begin your health education until you have made certain that there is an adequate supply of condoms at an affordable price. You

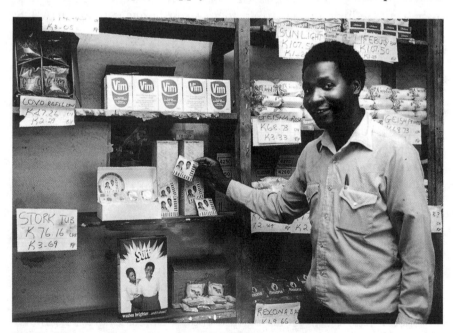

Fig 15. Social marketing of condoms through shops in Malawi

should try to use outlets such as shops, supermarkets, factories, bars and tea shops to make them easily accessible to all the key groups in the community.

Shopkeepers should be encouraged to display condoms prominently. Simple training should be provided for shopkeepers on how to reduce embarrassment for the purchaser and how to explain correct use of condoms. Health education programmes can provide support through radio promotions, posters for displaying outside shops and leaflets on how to use the condoms.

A useful approach is to use *social marketing* methods which gives careful attention to packaging, brand names, advertising, price and distribution. Social marketing programmes for condoms have been launched in many countries throughout the world. In Ghana and Jamaica condoms have been given the name 'Panther'. In Malawi the social marketing programme has launched the 'Protector' condoms which are available from bars and shops. In India a brand of condoms has been called 'Kama Sutra', after the famous Indian manual on sex.

Using effective communication methods

Mass media: radio, television and newspapers

Radio has several advantages as a communication medium for messages about AIDS. Many people listen to radio even in remote rural areas. Preparing radio programmes is not expensive. Radio messages can reach people who are illiterate and education can be combined with entertainment.

However, radio has some disadvantages. Radio messages tend to be general and cannot meet the needs of specific individuals or communities. You cannot ask for clarification if there is something that you do not understand or want to know more about. It is easy to spread panic and fear reactions through misunderstandings.

The fact that it is not possible to obtain clarification or check for misunderstanding makes radio most suited for simple messages: even so, it extremely important to test out the content of radio programmes to make sure that the message is clearly understood.

Radio can be used in many different ways in AIDS education. These are:

- interviews with local communities,
- panel discussions where health workers and others answer listener's questions,
- short spot announcements,

- magazine programmes with music and information,
- short dramas or AIDS education themes built into existing 'soap operas',
- competitions where the audience is asked to send in correct answers.

It is important to make the broadcasts as entertaining as possible with opportunities for audience feedback through letters and street interviews. If it is boring, people will not bother to listen. In northern Zambia the *Nshilakamona* radio drama was broadcast in the local language Bemba. It sought to capture the listener's attention through a dramatic portrayal of two families in Lusaka and their friends as they responded to problems of raising teenage children, friendships, making ends meet, their sex relations and AIDS

Serious thought needs to be given to the timing of broadcasts to suit the intended audience. During the day people may be at work but retired and unemployed persons or child carers may be at home. Late at night children will not be listening and this is a good time for reaching adults on their own. If you want to reach a large audience, you should broadcast at a time when many are listening such as just

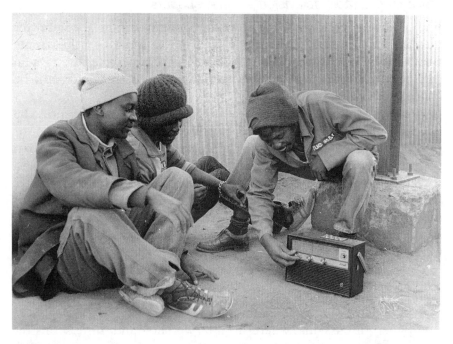

Figure 16. Radio is a good way of reaching large numbers of persons with simple information

before the news in the morning or evening. You should try to find out if there have been any audience surveys carried out which provide details of the listening times and favourite programmes of different groups in your community.

Television combines a spoken with a visual dimension so it is possible to show and demonstrate things visually. It can be entertaining and people show respect for and often believe what they see on television. A good example of the use of television is the *Soul City* programme in South Africa. It is a drama series that combines entertainment through situations where health issues are also brought out.

In many developing countries television and newspapers are still only received by a small section of the population. This can be an advantage if your aim is to reach the influential decision makers or urban people. But it is a disadvantage if you are trying to reach the poorer sections of the community or those living in rural areas.

A disadvantage with both radio and television is that there are often restrictions and government control on how freely sexual matters can be discussed on the mass media. It is usually easier to give frank information about sex face-to-face.

You may not be in a position to produce television or radio programmes but you can still use them. Look out for broadcasts on AIDS and follow them up with questions and discussions with your community. It is a good idea to make cassette recordings of any programmes on the radio or television and play them to groups of people at health centre waiting areas, schools or even workplaces. A voluntary agency in Madras, India, engaged local musicians and actors to produce cassettes for playing in clinics. Rap songs have been recorded on cassette to play to young people, cassettes on AIDS have been recorded to play through village loudspeakers in Thailand.

Printed materials: leaflets and posters

Leaflets are helpful for subjects such as sex when people may be too shy to ask. They are a useful reinforcement for individual and group sessions and serve as a reminder of the main points that you have made. Even if people cannot read they can ask others to read them aloud. Comic books have been successfully used to reach young people in an entertaining way. Many target groups described above such as children, youths, soldiers and sex workers will require leaflets that meet their very specific needs. It is also helpful to have a series of leaflets dealing with a range of topics, e.g. introducing AIDS, the use of a condom, information on the AIDS test and infection control practices for health care workers.

Many posters, booklets and leaflets have already been produced by a range of agencies. You might be able to use them directly in your health education work. However, they may not be relevant, either because of language, pictures or advice. You will probably have to produce your own locally appropriate materials. These do not have to be expensively produced to a sophisticated standard provided their content is relevant.

A useful starting point is to look at posters, booklets and leaflets produced in other programmes in your country and abroad. This will give you ideas on how you can adapt the ideas to your own situation. Use pictures to make them interesting and attractive. Make the language simple and try out draft versions with people from your target group to make sure that they are understood. Always include an address where people can write to or go to for further information. If you are translating from English take care to express the exact meaning in the local language. Give the leaflets out at talks or counselling sessions, leave them in public places and make them available on demand after a radio or television programme. Look out for opportunities to distribute them directly to households, e.g. in wage packets, voters registrations forms, electricity bills or rent statements.

A simple check list that you can use for testing out a leaflet is:

● Is it interesting to look at?

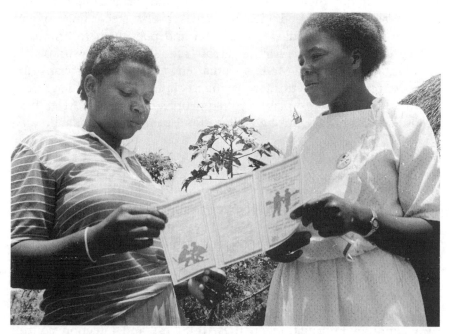

Figure 17. Using leaflets in AIDS education

- Does it contain relevant information for the target audience?
- Does it contain distracting irrelevant information?
- Is the language easy to read?
- Does it avoid complicated technical words?
- Is the advice presented realistic and feasible?
- Does it provide the specific information that the target audience actually *want* to know?
- Does it tell people where they can get further information from?

By themselves posters have little value. They are useful mainly to bring a topic to the attention of the community, reinforce a message that the people are receiving through other channels such as radio and person-to-person and provide a talking point for discussion. Examples of appropriate use of posters include: reinforcing the main theme of a radio campaign; a theme for a talk at a clinic; in a village to draw attention to a community meeting; and displayed outside a shop to say that condoms are available.

A good poster should have a very simple message and not try to say too much. It should be eye catching to gain attention through use of striking pictures, strong colours or interesting content. Posters should be displayed where your intended audience will pass them and see them. There is no point in just displaying them at clinics where they will only be seen by a small group of people. You will need to use different locations depending on the intended audience, e.g. young people, men, pregnant women, long distance drivers or soldiers. Do not leave them up for too long as people will become familiar with them and not notice them. In Johannesburg posters were displayed on city buses. Some programmes have used billboards. In Zambia they have even used the sides of waste bins on city streets!

Person-to-person AIDS education

Radio and television are good ways of reaching large sections of the population quickly with simple messages. However the important tasks of explaining the details of AIDS, providing specific advice on behaviour change, helping people to acquire skills (communication, decision making and manual), attitude change and empowerment can only really be carried out at a personal level.

We have already shown in Chapter 6 how face-to-face methods such as counselling can be used to explain more complex information, relieving anxieties and helping people make decisions about their personal sexual behaviour. Another form of person-to-person education is through small groups. Your role should be that of a facilitator, providing specific information where necessary, but promoting discussion and sharing of ideas between the participants.

It is important to start any individual or group teaching by finding out what your audience already knows and whether you have to meet any special needs or correct any misconceptions. People may be shy about asking questions in public. You can overcome this by putting them in pairs at the beginning to identify questions and concerns. Once they have discovered that others have similar questions and anxieties they will feel more confident about voicing these to the whole group. Another good method is to ask them to write questions out on pieces of paper that can be passed to the front or put anonymously into a box.

Role play

As described in the chapter on counselling, role play is a good technique for exploring difficult problems and attitudes as well as developing communication skills. One person can be assigned a particular role such as a young man, child, woman and another person is asked to give them advice, e.g. how to use a condom, what methods of sex are safe, how to avoid being infected with HIV in hospital. Others watch and at the end everybody comments on how the issues were handled and what improvements could have been made.

Drama and story telling

In Trinidad 30 villages were reached through a theatre production that showed the impact of AIDS on a single family. Extensive discussions were held after each performance. A mime and street theatre group *Jagran* ('awakening') has been performing at large scale events in North India watched by thousands of people.

There is a rich tradition of drama, story telling, songs and oral communication media in most communities that you can use in your health education. They are popular, well understood and good ways of involving people and creating interest. You should give local entertainers the basic background on AIDS and let them use their experience to adapt the message to their own words and music.

Puppets

Puppets are worth considering even if they are not familiar methods in your community. Some countries, e.g. India and Indonesia, have a rich heritage of puppet shows that are watched and enjoyed by people of all ages. AIDS is a serious subject and it is easy to offend people when discussing delicate issues surrounding sexual behaviour. Puppets are a way of raising sensitive issues without offending people.

It is possible to show actions and responses in puppets that would not be acceptable to show in a drama.

In South Africa, the 'Puppets Against AIDS' project has used large human size puppets to raise awareness about AIDS. Other programmes have used smaller puppets, e.g. glove puppets to entertain and inform the community.

There are cultures where puppets are watched by adults, however in other cultures puppets may be used only for entertaining children. Your community may feel reluctant to come to a puppet show and feel that they are being talked down to or treated like children. In practice though, if you can persuade them to come they will usually enjoy the puppets and find it worthwhile.

Visual aids and participatory learning

Can you make your talks more interesting? Well-chosen visual aids help to create interest, hold attention, put over difficult subjects and encourage learner participation. For example pictures of people in different social situations can be used to stimulate discussion on pressures to undertake high-risk sexual activities. Games and puzzles have been developed to provide entertaining and informative ways of learning information.

Learning aids do not have to be sophisticated and can be improvised from pictures from magazines or other sources. Examples of simple home-made learning aids are:

- pictures from film magazines to raise issues of sex in modern society;
- pictures of different types of social contact such as shaking hands, touching, eating food and kissing to show to groups to ask whether they transmit HIV;
- a model of a penis (bananas are good for this!) for demonstrating the putting on of condoms.

Video and audiocassettes

Video equipment may be available to make your own programmes. If not, you can still make use of the increasing number of well-produced information programmes on AIDS which may be available on loan from national or state AIDS control programmes. You can record programmes broadcast on radio or television. You should be selective in your choice of programmes. Make them relevant to your audience. You do not have to use the entire programme and can show just enough to trigger a discussion or stop it at appropriate points for discussions. Audio cassettes with music and slogans about AIDS have been played on buses in the African country of Zaire. Long-distance buses in some countries, e.g. India, have video players which could be used for AIDS education.

Advocacy

Advocacy is the process by which we seek to influence decision makers and those in power to take action. This is not easy as policy makers and politicians face pressure from many different directions. They will only take action if they feel that there is support from other politicians and the community. They will resist actions that are unpopular or will draw criticisms upon themselves.

As individuals, it is easy for us to feel powerless in the face of large organisations and political parties. We may also feel that we are opening ourselves to criticism and even abuse if we stand out and oppose government actions. The first step for effective advocacy is to find others who think like you and form a group to take action. Once a group has formed it can share responsibility for any decisions and individual members can be protected. You will have greater influence because there are more of you.

Once you have formed a group you should link up ('network') with other groups who share similar views inside your own country and internationally. This way you can exchange information and coordinate pressure. This might involve setting up local coalitions of groups who can join together on specific issues. Some of the actions that you could take include:

- Meet with journalists from newspapers, radio and television to give them information about AIDS and the need for policy change.
- Organise meetings, public events with visually striking photo opportunities, petitions and demonstrations to provide information and gain publicity, e.g. around special events such as World AIDS Day.
- Write to and meet policy makers to discuss the need for changes
- Draw the attention of public and policy makers to resolutions on AIDS from the United Nations and the World Health Assembly that, as member states, their country will have signed up to.
- Meet with professional organisations such as medical associations and trade unions to obtain their support for changes in policies for health and the workplace.
- Form networks with international organisations such as UNAIDS, International Council of AIDS Support Organisations and WHO.

Many AIDS education groups have found it worthwhile developing close links with journalists and producers. For example in Swaziland the National AIDS Committee has run seminars for journalists who have developed coordinated campaigns and produced guidelines for responsible coverage of AIDS in the media. Journalists and broadcasters are often looking for interesting material to include in their programmes and you should always send them details of your activities and give them sufficient advance notice to send a reporter. It is a good idea to prepare press releases in advance of any activity you carry out. A press release should explain what the activity is, when and where it will take place, why you are doing it and who you are (with a contact address and telephone number).

Evaluating your activities

Sexual behaviours are extremely difficult to change and are influenced by economic, social and cultural factors. What has worked in one situation may not succeed with another. A programme may not only fail to promote low risk behaviours, but can even make the situation worse by encouraging misunderstandings and panic responses. Can you find ways of evaluating the effects of your education to find out what works best with your community?

You should be realistic over what changes to look for in your evaluation. Changes in knowledge, understanding, awareness and belief might be achieved soon after your activity. However, changes in behaviour and health usually take longer. Some changes such as number of persons infected with HIV or using condoms properly are less suitable to use for evaluation because they are difficult to measure or get accurate data without an expensive survey. While your ultimate aim may be to reduce the number of cases of AIDS, this is not a useful measure for evaluation because it can take up to ten or more years for an infected person to develop clinical symptoms of AIDS.

Sexually transmitted infections can provide a useful indicator of whether the public is beginning to adopt safer sexual behaviour. Indicators of behaviour change that you could use for evaluation include the quantity of condoms distributed by clinics or sold at shops or bars. Surveys can be carried out to obtain data on the numbers of sexual partners and the use of condoms.

Surveys on delicate subjects such as sexual behaviour have to be carried out very carefully to ensure that the information collected represents what is really going on. The most reliable information often comes from small-scale studies with individuals and groups. In this kind of study, called 'qualitative research,' you put time and effort into gaining the confidence and participation of the community and let them express in their own words their feelings about your educational activities.

It is a good idea to carry out a *short-term evaluation* fairly soon after the activity and a *follow-up evaluation* 1–2 years afterwards to look for long-term changes. In evaluating your work you can ask the following questions.

- How many people did you reach?
- Did you reach those at highest risk?
- Did it lead to improvements in knowledge and/or behaviour?
- Were there unexpected benefits/disadvantages?
- What did the intended audience think about the programme?
- Were the benefits worth the effort and expense involved?
- How could the education be improved?
- Were there any unusual factors that led to success/failure?
- Would the activity work with a different community?

Sharing your experiences with others – building a global movement

Be prepared to share the findings from your evaluations with others as this is the only way to build up a body of knowledge and experience. Do not feel embarrassed about telling others of your failures as this might stop others from making the same mistakes. Your National AIDS Control Programme will always be glad to hear about your work and how they can provide support. At the end of this book there is a list of international newsletters that are always interested in your work. One of the most exciting developments since the last edition of this book has been the establishment of the global network of computers that make up the Internet. Many organizations such as UNAIDS, WHO, UNICEF and Centers for Disease Control now have Web sites details of which are provided below. These provide valuable information on AIDS and a point of contact and information exchange. The growth of e-mail as a cheap form of communication makes it possible to network across the world, form discussion groups about treatment, prevention and global action. You can now keep up with the fast-moving scene of prevention and treatment. More important, by sharing your experiences, you become part of a global community in the fight against AIDS.

Further information

Books

Adam, G. & Harford, M. (2000) *Radio and HIV/AIDS: Making a Difference: A guide for radio practitioners, health workers and donors.* Media Action International and UNAIDS, Geneva.

Adler, M. (1997) *ABC of AIDS* (4th edition). British Medical Journal Publishing Group, London.

Adler, M. (1999) *ABC of Sexually Transmitted Diseases* (4th edition). British Medical Journal Publishing Group, London.

Crofton, J., Horne, N. & Miller, F. (1999) *Clinical Tuberculosis* (2nd edition). Macmillan, London and Oxford.

Gordon, G. (1999) *Choices – a guide for young people.* Macmillan Education, London and Oxford

Gordon, G. (1999) *A Narrow Escape. (*A reader for schools which explains AIDS through a story of a young girl's narrow escape.)Macmillan's Living Health Series, London and Basingstoke.

Hubley, J.H. (1993) *Communicating Health – An action guide to health education and health promotion.* Macmillan Publishers, London and Oxford.

Jackson, H. (1992) *AIDS: Action Now – Information, prevention and support in Zimbabwe.* AIDS Counselling Trust, PO Box 7225, Harare, Zimbabwe.

Ng'weshemi, J.Z., Boerma, J.T., Bennet, J., & Schapink, D. (eds) (1997) *HIV Prevention and AIDS Care in Africa – A district level approach.* Kit Press, Royal Tropical Institute, Amsterdam, The Netherlands.

Williams, G. (series editor) *Strategies for Hope –* A series of case study booklets and video programmes which aims to promote informed, positive thinking and practical action. No 1 *From Fear to Hope,* No 2 *Living Positively with AIDS,* No 3 *AIDS Management,* No 4 *Meeting AIDS with Compassion,* No 5 *AIDS Orphans,* No 6 *The Caring Community,* No 7 *All Against AIDS,* No 8 *Work Against AIDS – workplace initiatives in Zimbabwe,* No 9 *Candles of Hope,* No 10 *Filling the Gaps,* No 11 *Broadening the Front,* No 12 *A Common Cause,* No. 13 *Youth-to-Youth,* No 14 *Under the Mpundu Tree,* No 15 *Open Secret.* Published by Strategies of Hope and available from Teaching-aids At Low Cost (see address below).

UNAIDS and WHO publications

Impact of HIV and Sexual Health Education on the Sexual Behaviour of Young People (1997). UNAIDS.

Summary Booklet of Best Practices (1999, and see updates). UNAIDS.
HIV in Pregnancy: a review (1999). WHO/UNAIDS.
AIDS Home Care Handbook (1993). WHO.
(A wide range of useful publications are available free from UNAIDS either from their
Intenet Web site or on request from their address – see below.)

Newsletters
(Free to persons from developing countries)

AIDS Action. Healthlink, 1 London Bridge St., London SE1 9SG, UK.
HIV/AIDS Action in Developing Countries. Newsletter from the European Union,
European Commission, (SCR E) Rue Belliard 28 – B 28.6/146, Brussels, Belgium.
Population Reports. Population Information Programme, Johns Hopkins University,
527 St. Paul Place, Baltimore, MD 21202, USA.
Sexual Health Exchange. Royal Tropical Institute, Mauritskade 631092 AD Amsterdam,
The Netherlands (published in association with the Southern African AIDS
information Service)

Teaching materials

Slide sets: *HIV Infection – Virology and Transmission* (HIVV) describes virology,
immunology, epidemiology and transmission of HIV; *HIV Infection – Clinical
Manifestations* (HIVC) clinical case definition and clinical manifestations of HIV
infection in adults and children in Africa; *HIV Infection – Clinical Manifestations in
Asia* (HICA) Clinical case definition and clinical manifestations of HIV infection
in adults in the Asian and Pacific region; *HIV Infection in Children* (HIVP) provides
an overview of HIV infection in children including epidemiology, transmission,
diagnosis, clinical manifestations, management and community issues; *HIV
Infection – Prevention and Counselling* (HIVE) discusses problems of prevention of
transmission of infection and possible health education approaches. *Peer Group
Education in AIDS and STD Programmes* (HIVM) introduces the concept of peer
education through an example from Malawi with sex workers and truck drivers.
Sexually Transmitted Diseases (STR) shows how to recognise and treat common
sexually transmitted diseases. These slide sets are intended for medical and other
experienced health workers and are modestly priced according to mounting type.
Stepping Stones. Manuals and video. A complete package for running educational
workshops for community members on HIV/AIDS. Published by Strategies for
Hope and available from TALC.
Sexually Transmitted Diseases Pack: A pack of picture cards which show how to
recognize and treat common STDSs.
AIDS Educational Game. A board game which provides a way for children, young
people and adults to learning about HIV/AIDS and sexual health.

All teaching materials available from Teaching-aids At Low Cost, P.O. Box 49, St
Albans, Herts, AL1 5TX, UK.

Useful addresses

Healthlink Worldwide (formerly called ARHTAG), Cityside, 40 Alder Street, London E1 1EE, UK. e-mail: info@healthlink.org.uk

Centre for Communication Programmes, Johns Hopkins School of Hygiene and Public Health, Johns Hopkins University, 62 North Broadway, Baltimore, Maryland 21205, USA. e-mail: webadmin@jhuccp.org

Centre de Formation pour la Promotion de la Sante, BP 1800, Kangu, Mayumbe, Zaire

Child-to-Child Trust, Institute of Education, 20 Bedford Way, London WC1H 0AL, UK. e-mail: c.scotchmer@ioe.ac.uk

Teaching-aids At Low Cost (TALC), PO Box 49, St Albans, Herts AL1 4TX, UK. e-mail: talc@talcuk.org

UNICEF, 3 United Nations Plaza, New York, NY 10017, USA. e-mail: netmaster@unicef.org

UNESCO. Unit for Cooperation with UNICEF and WFP, UNESCO, 7 Place de Fontenoy, 75700 Paris, France

UNAIDS, 20, avenue Appia, CH-1211 Geneva 27, Switzerland. e-mail unaids@unaids.org

Useful Web sites on the Internet

Agencies

European Commission (www.europa.eu.int/comm/development/aids)
UNAIDS (www.unaids.org/)
UNICEF (www.unicef.org/)
WHO (www.who.int/)

Networks

ACT-UP (Activist organization – AIDS Coalition to Unleash Power) (www.actupny.org/)
The Global Network of people living with HIV/AIDS (www.gnpplus.net)
International Council of AIDS Service Organizations (ICASO) (www.icaso.org/)
International Gay and Lesbian Human Rights Commission (IGLHRC) (www.iglhrc.org/)

Resources

AEGIS (www.aegis.com) – research data
AIDS Law Project (www.hri.ca/partners/alp/index.html)
Anti-retroviral newsletter: (www.who.int/health-topics/std.htm)
AVERT (www.avert.org) – general information
Condom CD-ROM (www.jhuccp.org/popline/condom.stm) – details on condoms
Congress of South African Trade Unions, COSATU (www.cosatu.org.za)
Drum Beat – Communications newsletter (www.comminit.com)
Oneworld (www.oneworld.org) – useful NGOs on development
Johns Hopkins Communication project: (www.jhuccp.org)
SEA–AIDS (www.unaidsapict.inet.co.th/) (AIDS in Asia)
Strategies for Hope (www.actionaid.org/stratshope)

Details of other useful organisations can be found in the links section of the UNAIDS Internet Web site

Index